HUNGRY FOR HEALTH, STARVED FOR TIME

The Busy Person's Guide to Harmonious Health

SUZY HARMON
your greatest wealth is health

HUNGRY FOR HEALTH, STARVED FOR TIME
The Busy Person's Guide to Harmonious Health

Copyright ©2016 Susan Harmon All rights reserved.

All rights reserved. No part of this book may be reproduced in any form or by any electronic or mechanical means, including information storage and retrieval systems, without permission in writing from the author. For information, contact Suzy Harmon at (harmonioushealth@sbcglobal.net).

The content of this book is for general instruction only. Each person's physical, emotional, and spiritual condition is unique. The instruction in this book is not intended to replace or interrupt the reader's relationship with a physician or other professional. Please consult your doctor for matters pertaining to your specific health and diet.

To contact the author, visit
www.SuzyHarmoniousHealth.com

ISBN - 10: 1-944134-04-2
ISBN - 13: 978-1-944134-04-4

Printed in the United States of America

SPECIAL THANKS:

Thanks to Deb Silverthorn for the back cover photography.

Thanks to the team at Promoting Natural Health, to Amie Olson, Creative Director, for the fabulous cover design and book layout, and to Amanda Filippelli, Editor-in-Chief, for her amazing edits, proofing, and for helping me convey my message and my passion. It was a pleasure and an honor to work with all of you.

Acknowledgements

To my IIN community, you are my tribe. It is with all of you that I started my health journey. Together we are changing the health of the world, one health coaching client at a time. Thank you to Joshua Rosenthal for this incredible movement you started, and to Lindsey Smith and all the book course moderators. Your support made this book dream come true.

To Bradley, my oldest son, who, even at age four, listened to me preaching about the dangers of "hydrogenated oil." I love that you took my advice back then, and are still asking for it today.

To Zach, when you call me from college for advice on what to eat, I bet you don't know that I keep you on the phone and give you way more information than you need just so I can hear your voice a little longer. Well, maybe you know, but thank you for building my confidence in my coaching skills, and for sharing my cooking videos with the frat guys. I remember how hard it was to eat healthy in college and I applaud your efforts.

To Lindsay, thank you for editing my HarmonHealth Instagram photos and sharing them with your friends so I would have followers in the beginning! I am sorry for those recipes I was testing that didn't turn out so perfect. I know the amount of "junk food" in the house has practically disappeared since the boys left home, and the transition has been hard for you. Thank you for understanding how important healthy living is, for believing in what I am doing, and for giving it a try.

To Mom, thank you for always believing in me, and for always seeing the positive side of everything. It is from you that I learned to cook with love, and how important optimism is to one's health.

To all my girlfriends, you fill my life with wonderful primary food and are there to enjoy the secondary food with me (with a little wine), and I love you all.

To my clients, thank you for your confidence in me, and for the courage to make changes in your nutrition and lifestyle habits. It is because of all of you that I keep plugging away and coaching and doing what I love to do.

To my family and friends, I have learned from all of you the importance of having strong, caring relationships in life, and that support fuels me every day to wake up and do what I do.

And finally, to my amazing husband, Andy, you are everything…no, really, literally, you are everything—my PR Team, my ad agency, my tech support. Thank you for your constant support always, and for saying, "I think you NEED to write this book." I can't wait to share many more healthy life "experiences" yet to come with you. I love you, dude.

Dedication

I dedicate this book to my father, Earl Sussman, who I miss and think of every day. I thank him for filling my life with the gift of happy memories. Dad inspired my first career as a CPA, and later inspired me to look inward to begin my own health journey, which has led to my new career as a health coach.

I will never forget spending a beautiful fall Saturday with my dad at Mohonk Mountain House in New York's Hudson Valley. As we stared out at the top of a tall hill overlooking the beautiful fall foliage and the sun sparkling on the water, he taught me one of life's greatest lessons. He told me to take in the view and remember it, and to *"never forget the big picture and what really matters."* So often, when I feel overwhelmed or unsure of myself, I pause, close my eyes, and remember that beautiful view and the warmth of his arm on my shoulder, and suddenly, everything falls into perspective.

I know he would be proud of this book and of my desire to help people create Harmonious Health in their lives.

Contents

My Story—In a New York Minute 9
Introduction 17
How to Use This Book 21

1. Healthy Home Environment 25
Create a Sacred Space 27
Sleep Like a Baby 31
Bring the Outdoors Inside 35
Change Your Tune 38
Clear up the Clutter, Beat the Clock 40

2. Healthy Eating 43
Eat Mindfully 45
Don't Bite off More than You Can Chew 49
Quick Switches 52
Drink Up: Keep Your Head Above Water 59
Eat with the Seasons 61
Food and Finances 64

3. Healthy Body 69
Brush Your Skin 71
Ditch Your All-or-Nothing Attitude 73
Give Your Stomach Acid a Boost 76
Health for the Tip of your Tongue 81
Read Your Personal Care Product Labels 84
Who Ya Gonna Call? ...Stress Busters 87

4. Healthy Cooking   93
Is There Prana in Your Food?   96
Experiment with New Tastes   99
Simple Meals in next to No Time   103
Fail to Plan or Plan to Fail   107
Invest in Some Kitchen Gadgets & Use Them   110

5. Healthy Mind   115
No Time to Think? Use a Journal   118
Remember to Breathe   121
Focus on Your Primary Food   123
Take Time for Nature   128
Give Your Cravings the Time of Day   131
Meal Planning   135

Cut to the Chase   141
About the Author   145

MY STORY
In a New York Minute

I am not a scientist and I am not medically trained. In fact, I spent over twenty years working in the corporate world in New York City as a CPA doing financial audits, writing accounting policy manuals, and preparing financial statements for large corporate clients. **So, why am I writing a book about health, and why should you care?**

Maybe you are working in a career filled with success and excitement, or you are a busy parent at home taking care of young kids. For the most part, you are enjoying your career and your life, but like me, you are busy! Juggling the demands of a family, your job, taking care of a home, or perhaps aging parents can be overwhelming. Sometimes you feel exhausted by all of the roles you play and by all of the responsibilities calling for your attention, and the thought of adding anything to your plate, like new health habits, seems impossible. We want to be good enough, attractive enough, thin enough, smart enough, reply to emails fast enough, but enough is enough!!

That was my experience several years ago when my family and I relocated to Dallas, Texas from New York. What began as just a few sporadic days of feeling overloaded and tired turned into an almost constant state of discomfort. I began to notice some slight weight gain around my mid-section, aches and pains in my shoulders, neck and legs, thinning hair, skin breakouts, difficulty concentrating (or what I call foggy brain), and as I would get in bed, I often felt engulfed by a sense of overwhelm and could not slow my thoughts down. Clearly my health and wellbeing were suffering, but with no free time to spare, I was at a loss as to what I should do.

I was eating pretty well (or so I thought), and I would fit in exercise when I could, but I did not have time to be one of those crazy health freaks. Sometimes, I would spot those people (the health freaks, as I called them) out running, or at the grocery store with weird health foods in their shopping carts. Other times I could spot them in an elevator, on an airplane, or in line at the bank. They were the ones who stood tall, the whites of their eyes shining, and they looked energetic, calm, full of life, and most of all…happy. During this period of time, when I was feeling achy and foggy, I would often gaze at the health freaks and think, "They must not have jobs. They must have loads of leisure time and money to devote to being healthy." I was getting older and I thought maybe this is just the kind of "stuff" that happens to your body as you get older, but then I started noticing that a lot of these healthy, happy folks were way older than me, so that shot down that theory. What was their secret? How did they live so healthy? They seemed so serene, it must be so easy for them.

Some days I would feel so frustrated about my muffin top, my achy body, and think, "What more could I need to do? I am maxed out. I can't add another thing to my plate." I was under a misconception that I did not have time to be healthy, at least certainly not during the busy workweek. I thought, "Busy people like me can't take hours of time out of their day to cook healthy meals or exercise during the workweek." Healthy living was meant for the two days during the weekend, when life was a little slower. Healthy living was meant for the rich and famous who had loads of extra time and money to hire chefs and personal trainers, not for ordinary people like me. I was wrong.

Some days I tried to get up thirty minutes early during the week to go to a class at the gym, but the thought of that loud aerobics class at the gym did not always lure me out of bed. I have since learned that the loud and crowded class was not what my body needed on those mornings and that is why I could not get motivated. Now I start my day with yoga poses and light stretches or a peaceful run outside, alone with my thoughts. I am able to motivate myself to get up thirty minutes earlier much more consistently because I have connected with the type of movement that is right for my particular body type and my mindset, and what time of day works best for my body to exercise. Sometimes I wanted to cook a super healthy, beautiful, special dinner for the family during the week, like a hearty soup or a stew filled with amazing vegetables, but who had the time to stand around chopping vegetables on a weekday evening when the kids needed to be driven to French horn lessons, and soccer practice, or when I had a PTA meeting to attend? I have now learned how just a small amount of weekend prep can allow me to cook beautiful, healthy meals all week long, effortlessly.

I came to realize that being healthy does not have to be time consuming, it does not have to involve bouncing from doctor to doctor. It just involves a greater awareness of what type of movement and foods our bodies need to run efficiently. When we identify and connect with our individual body's needs as opposed to a preconceived idea of what "healthy" living looks like, the obstacle of time diminishes. Today, I actually laugh when people tell me I am one of those "health freaks" because my everyday life is so different than how I imagined those healthy people lived. I do not have loads of free leisure time and money or no job, but I have found a way to live an active, well-nourished lifestyle, simply and easily. When we choose exercise we enjoy, that makes us feel rejuvenated and energized when we are through, we are more likely to turn it into a habit we stick with. When we feel a pressure to be a jogger, but we hate jogging, we can't find the time to fit it in. When we think a healthy dinner must include a plate full of kale, but we hate kale, we think, "I just don't have the time for all of that intensive work." When we do not understand how the common foods we have been eating our entire lives are causing detrimental effects on our body and mind, we accept our tired, overweight, moody selves and chalk it up to age. So how did I get there, and what was the final motivating factor?

When I lost my dad to a battle with lung cancer, I started opening up to the various people in my life in my roles as a wife, a mother, a daughter, a sister, a friend, a PTA member, a community volunteer, and was amazed to hear how many people suggested taking prescription medications which were helping them with anxiety or insomnia. So I met with doctors who suggested anxiety medications and ADHD medications. They suggested the ADHD medications because I answered ten questions, the gist of which were, "Do you think about more than one thing at a time?" What busy person would not say yes to that? But these medications only served to curb my appetite and prevented me from listening to my body and what it needed. They caused me to either oversleep on the weekends or to not sleep enough during the week, they dehydrated me, and they did very little to improve my symptoms.

After a couple years of this, I became fed up with taking pills that were not doing a lot to help me, but did not know where else to turn. One evening, while I was on the internet, I learned about a school called the Institute for Integrative Nutrition (IIN). They offered a health coach training program that seemed to call my name, but I hesitated to enroll and step out of my comfort zone. I thought, "What business does a CPA have studying about nutrition and wellbeing?" That following week, my dear childhood friend lost her husband to an unexplained health problem just shy of his 50th birthday. I thought about this dear friend of mine, about my dad who I lost a few years prior, about my own health issues, and about so many other friends and family members who were suffering with health problems and illnesses, or who had lost loved ones to disease. My urge to enroll in IIN became even stronger, but I still felt unsure.

So what do you do when you are a fifty-year-old woman and you cannot decide what to do? I called my mom, who I am lucky enough to have in my life!

My mom said, "You do not need to begin a new career. You can just learn and acquire this great information to support yourself, your family, and your friends."

My husband and my three kids were supporters of the idea as well. At that point, I realized that I could either wake up every day and pop pills that affected my appetite, my energy, and basically created new symptoms to mask the ones that I was trying to treat, or I could step way out of my comfort zone and see if I could learn to heal myself and improve my energy by creating a healthier, happier life through a new approach. So, despite my fear, I enrolled in nutrition school. I felt inspired to learn what I could, to do what I could to feel better, and to improve my health and the health of those I loved.

While I expected to learn a bit about food, nutrition, and healthy living, I never expected that my year in nutrition school would be such a life changing experience. During that year, I continued to work in the accounting field while I studied in the evenings. I think I was able to find the time to study because as I began to incorporate what I was learning in class into my daily life, I noticed that many of my uncomfortable symptoms began to diminish and eventually, completely disappear. I had improved energy and less aches and pains. My anxiety and brain fog diminished, and I gradually reduced and then removed all prescription medications from my life. I am now, happily, medication free. As I continued to feel better and better, I wanted to spend more and more time learning and studying. My hair got thicker and my skin cleared up, my clothes fit better, and I felt fabulous. I felt so wonderful that I wanted to share what I learned in nutrition school with as many people as I could. So I gradually cut back on my accounting work and began a new career as a health coach, hoping to spread the ripple effect of what I had learned. Living a healthy lifestyle felt so incredible, and I was shocked to learn that it was not "freaky" at all, but actually simple, doable, and life changing. Creating a healthier lifestyle is easier than most people think and not nearly as time consuming as people imagine. **That is why I am writing this book about health.**

In the hustle of life, raising a family, making a living, our society is very quick to turn to prescription medications and poor food choices as ways of comforting ourselves and calming our stress. It seems like the perfect quick fix. While I also believe there are many people who greatly benefit from these prescriptions, I feel very strongly that there are thousands of people out there, just like me, who could be healing themselves through a more holistic approach if only they had someone to help them and guide them. There is a strong need for health coaches in our world today because doctors are too busy to hold people's hands and walk them through the steps necessary to reduce their stress, improve their diets, cook more, shop healthier, and hold them accountable on a weekly basis, as I do in my health coaching program. Now I want to share some of the tools I use in my health coaching program with you so you, too, can make small, easy, and gradual changes to your daily habits like I did, and feel fabulous. These health habits are not complicated, difficult, or terribly time consuming, yet they can have a profound effect on your health. I hope you will try to implement the ones that resonate with you and begin to notice yourself feeling more vibrant, full of life, happier, and healthier.

I understand the challenges you are facing when you are trying to live a healthy AND busy life, and I want to share how you can overcome them by incorporating simple routines into your week that will dramatically improve how you feel. You do not need to find more hours in the day, you just need to be willing to take small simple steps forward every day to learn and incorporate. I am so passionate about teaching people how easy this can be, and I hope my passion will inspire you also as you read my book. Take it slow, one small action step at a time, and before you know it, this will all be habit for you and you will feel amazing and harmoniously healthy. Read on. Your healthiest, best self is only pages away.

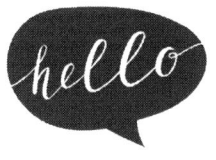

INTRODUCTION

The busy corporate financial world in New York City was always very exciting to me. Whether I was working for the accounting firm of Laventhol & Horwath, traveling to different clients and learning about their companies, or working internally in the corporate accounting departments of amazing companies such as Paramount Pictures or Young & Rubicam Advertising, I found it thrilling.

I particularly remember budget presentation days, whether on Madison Avenue, Columbus Circle, or any other location, as being a bit overwhelming. I sat in countless budget meetings over the twenty plus years of my financial career. We would sit with high-level corporate executives, present our analyses, and often worked late into the evening, discussing the future health of the company, planning expenses, projecting cash flow, and ensuring that the future of the company was healthy and stable. Sometimes I would just sit back and look around the conference table at the endless cans of diet soda, coffee cups, bags of chips, doughnuts, and bowls of candy and wonder if anyone else saw the irony. I thought to myself, "No one is going to be alive to enjoy all of this financial success if everyone keeps eating and drinking all of this crap." I wanted to stand on the conference table and scream, "Don't you people realize that your greatest wealth is your health?!" That has since become the tagline for my coaching program.

Inertia often rules the thought process of busy boardroom executives. They get into a pattern of neglecting their health because they think they do not have time. These executives can put together virtually any business deal if they are determined to do so. It is not that they can't find the time to focus on their wellbeing, they could do anything they want. It is that they have been neglecting their health for so long that it has become a habit. So many corporate executives think they have no time for their health, but these are the leaders setting an example for their employees. When they are too busy or too resistant to suggestions about changing their habits and they ignore the importance of their health, they allow their health to suffer and they inadvertently send a message to their employees that can negatively affect the culture in a company. The result creates an organization filled with low energy, out of shape employees who are unmotivated because they feel like crap.

While you might not be a business owner, you are the CEO of your busy life, and your health is truly the most important possession you own. I always ask my clients, "What is your 'why?' Why do you want to be healthy? Why should you care about your health?" Most people tell me their "why" consists of their children or their loved ones, and they want to be around for many years to enjoy them. Often, when you can get very clear on your "why," it becomes much easier to commit to addressing your health and what you need to do to improve it. Maybe your "why" is a hobby you enjoy or maybe your "why" really is your career because you find it deeply meaningful and rewarding. Whatever it is, I urge you now to really stop and think about how you would feel if something happened to your health that would prevent you from achieving your "why." When you get very clear on this, it becomes a motivator to help you break out of the inertia of feeling like you have no time, like you have too much stress, you lack focus, or that you have limited resources, and to make a commitment to address your health right now.

For those of you working hard to achieve success, but who feel frustrated because you are starting to realize that you are so often ignoring your health, you can do both. The two are not mutually exclusive. Whether your definition of success is raising your children, being successful in your job, having a comfortable home, taking vacations with your family, or doing fun activities with your friends, there is a way to work toward this goal without neglecting yourself. None of it is worthwhile in the long term if you are jeopardizing your health. Now is the time to stop ignoring your health in pursuit of wealth.

I am always happy to work with and help clients who have survived a health scare, or who have been shaken by the residual fear of seeing a loved one survive a health scare. Don't wait until this is you. Take steps now to get started on your new health journey. Can you hear me screaming like I wanted to in all of those conference rooms? **Your greatest wealth is your health.**

Today, I know that the best thing we could have done in those crazy late night budget meetings would've been to pause, do some deep breathing, stand up and stretch, open some windows and let in some fresh air, ditch the sugar and caffeine and swap it for some healthy green smoothies or snack on some whole fruits, veggies, nuts and seeds. These are exactly some of the things I teach time starved individuals and corporate groups to do in order to maintain their greatest resource—their health. Read on to learn more about how to protect your greatest asset, your health.

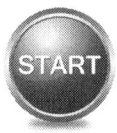

HOW TO USE THIS BOOK

This book is a condensed sample of many of the topics I work on with clients in my health coaching program. I will break down the habits of healthy living for everyday people into five different categories:

Home Environment Habits
Eating Habits
Body Care Habits
Cooking Habits
Habits for the Mind

I often notice people get very focused on just one of these areas. They try to be "perfect" in this one area of focus. What I learned on my own personal health journey is that this type of an approach can be very risky. At one point, I got so focused on my eating habits that I almost developed *orthorexia,* which is an unhealthy obsession with eating healthy food.

A better approach is to be a little imperfect in every area, but consistently take small steps forward in each of the five areas every week. As you progress, you will start to feel better and realize that when you cannot accomplish something one day in one area, you can compensate in another area. For example, I might have to miss a weekday workout, but I can get home, do some deep breathing exercises, and then cook a delicious whole food meal for my family with food I prepped over the weekend. Eventually, you will look at your life and realize you are in harmony and feeling balanced in all five of these important areas, that you feel great, and that you are achieving harmonious health.

The most lasting results are obtained when people just take very small, consistent steps on a daily basis. Each week, choose one habit from each chapter to focus on and work on it during that week. Keep in mind your "WHY?" on a weekly basis. When you focus on why you want to be healthy instead of the results you want, it will help keep you in the game and motivated. People often give up after a few weeks of making better eating or exercise choices because they do not see or feel the results they desire immediately. I always remind my clients that it took them a lifetime of habits to build the body they live in, so they cannot expect to change that in just a few weeks. However, taking small steps forward every day will definitely start to add up, and soon these steps will become new habits that you do not even have to think about. When that starts to happen is when you will slowly begin to feel the change. It is similar to the theory of compound interest. Investing a small amount, even just a penny a day, might not feel like much after just a few weeks, but over time, consistently performing this investment habit can add up to a sizeable amount. In a similar way, taking these small steps forward each day to develop new health habits can add up to wonderful health.

I wish you joy, happiness, and contentment on your harmonious health journey, and the strength to stay motivated to achieve your "why."

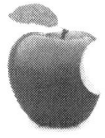

1

Healthy Home Environment

"He is happiest, be he king or peasant, who finds peace in his home."

- Johann Wolfgang von Goethe

If your home is not filled with positive and loving relationships, nourishing food, a healthy, clean, clutter-free environment, and a comfortable place to rest and renew your body, it is hard to find peace in your home. Think about your childhood and the home you grew up in. What memories do you have? Our home environment is a special place where we create memories, learn, nourish ourselves, bond with others, cleanse our bodies, and rest. Your home environment can have a profound impact on your health and your life.

In this chapter, I discuss the importance of changing your home environment to help you to feel more at ease, more productive, even better organized and focused. Taking time to "tune up your home environment" can make your busy life and schedule less stressful and more manageable.

To create a healthy home environment where you feel at peace, happy, and healthy, you do not need to own a mansion. The tips I share below do not cost massive amounts of money, but they can have a massive impact on your health and healing transformation if you implement them in your home. Focus on them by addressing one or two of them over a weekend until you have them implemented.

CREATE A SACRED SPACE IN YOUR HOME

Of course it would be wonderful if we had time in our daily routine to designate a place for everything in our home and to return each item there immediately after using it. But let's face it, life happens, and that is not always possible. We try our best, but children's needs must be tended to, carpool duty calls, an urgent work phone call comes in, the list goes on. Most of us just do not have adequate time to keep our home environment in pristine condition all the time, unless of course, you have the funds to hire a maid or assistant to clean up after you.

What I have learned is that if I dedicate one area of my home as a "sacred space" and do my best to keep that area as perfectly organized as possible, it creates a wonderful refuge for me at the end of the day. The benefit to my mind and body of having this sacred space is so great that it keeps me motivated to keep it tidy and neat. Since I do not really have an extra room in my home for that, I have designated a corner of my bedroom for this purpose. In that space I have a comfy chair, a side table with pretty flowers, some writing journals with my favorite pens, scented candles, and my new favorite hobby—some adult coloring books and colored pencils. I keep a special hand cream there to use while I relax.

Knowing that I can rely on this spot to welcome me and energize me at the end of the day is a great feeling. Admittedly, if you feel short on time, this probably sounds like just another "to do" to add to your schedule, but take a moment to consider this: While it is true that spending time socializing with others is good for us, spending time alone is important to our health because it allows us to improve our focus and creativity. It helps raise our awareness and understanding of our own thought processes, something known as metacognition. According to the Boston Globe Article, *The Power of Lonely,*

> "One ongoing Harvard study indicates that people form more lasting and accurate memories if they believe they're experiencing something alone. Another indicates that a certain amount of solitude can make a person more capable of empathy towards others. And while no one would dispute that too much isolation early in life can be unhealthy, a certain amount of solitude has been shown to help teenagers improve their moods and earn good grades in school."

(Neyfakh, Leon. The Power of Lonely: What We Do Better Without People Around. The Boston Globe. Boston Globe Media Partners, LLC. 2016. Web.)

Improved creativity, focus, awareness of our thoughts, and empathy toward others will often help us to solve the problems we are most struggling with just by the simple act of being in solitude and doing nothing. Being alone in your thoughts allows you time to renew yourself, and fuels and empowers you to take your health into your own hands. Allowing time for this on a daily basis will empower you to gain more ownership of your everyday nutrition and lifestyle choices.

After dinner, I will snuggle with my favorite blanket in this spot with a cup of herbal tea and let it rejuvenate me. I shut my door and usually enjoy the silence, but sometimes I will play some soft music. Having this time alone helps me sort through the issues of the day and unwind before I get into bed. Creating this sacred space has allowed me to pay attention to how my body is feeling, to notice any aches or pains, and to understand on a more regular basis what my body is telling me. For example, sometimes I notice I am dehydrated or that I need to stretch, and I can give my body what it needs. It is very important to learn how to listen to your body, and creating a safe and comfortable sacred space for yourself, away from the distractions of TV or other electronics, can provide you with the perfect way to do this.

Where can you set up a sacred space for yourself in your home? Give it a try and you will be amazed at how much you begin to look forward to relaxing in this space at the end of a long day. A sacred space is also a very simple, inexpensive, and effective way to prevent our bodies from suffering from the effects that, unattended to, long-term stress can have on our health. Start creating your sacred space today!

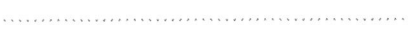

Harmonious Tip:

Be on the lookout for a small, inexpensive end-table to put in your sacred space where you can place a book, cup of tea or a candle. This will really make your space feel like it is your own. Once you get this set up schedule time, maybe just 5 minutes to start, to sit in that space and allow youself permission to unwind, relax, and practice self-care. This is one of the greatest gifts we can give ourselves. The payback will be obvious as you start to feel better and begin to accomplish more.

SLEEP LIKE A BABY

When Dr. Rubin Naiman spoke at the Institute for Integration Nutrition about the interface between nutrition with sleep and dreams, I was amazed to learn how much eating impacts sleep and how sleep impacts our eating, metabolism, and weight. He discussed how sleep is one of the cornerstones of good health. When we get a good night's sleep, our thoughts are clearer and our mood is more stable during the day.

Our society does not value sleep. I notice that people seem to feel a sense of pride when they discuss how busy they are and how little sleep they get. We need to renegotiate our relationship with sleep and begin to value its importance to our health.

In order to get proper sleep, it is important that we have good sleep hygiene, which refers to the habits that are conducive to sleeping well on a regular basis. When I began to understand how sleep deprivation was affecting my health, I developed a greater appreciation for finding ways to achieve good sleep, and lots of it. Often, my ruminating thoughts, fears, and worries would flare up just as I got into bed and would keep me awake for hours. When I decided to trade in that time spent worrying between midnight and 1:00am, and instead invest time in some sleep hygiene rituals an hour before bed, I found myself being much more productive and effective during the daytime. This improved productivity helped me to better navigate through my busy schedule, and help free up a little extra time each day. This led to a greater desire to continue practicing my sleep hygiene rituals.

One sleep hygiene ritual I now incorporate into my evening a few times a week includes taking a warm bubble bath filled with a calming essential oil such as lavender. The scent relaxes my body and mind, which has helped me to halt the ruminating thoughts when I get into bed. Often, I add Epson salt to the bath, which contains magnesium. When we are under a lot of stress, and eating a poor diet, often we become deficient in magnesium, so by bathing in an Epson salt bath, we can restore our magnesium levels as the minerals are absorbed through our skin. This will help our central nervous system to relax and can soothe body aches and pains, which all will lead to a better night's sleep as well as help us to fall asleep more easily. On the nights when you just don't have the ability to take a full bath, use a warm washcloth and gently massage it all over your body to help you unwind. The warmth of the washcloth helps to raise your body temperature, and then, as you dry off and dress in pajamas, you start to relax as your body cools off. When our body temperature starts to drop, our metabolic activity naturally starts to decrease, so our breathing slows down, our blood pressure drops, and we start to feel drowsy.

Another great sleep hygiene ritual you can try is called progressive muscle relaxation. Sometimes I cannot even get through my entire body muscles because I fall asleep while I am doing it. I like to start the exercise at the top of my body and work my way down. You start by tensing each muscle group and then relaxing it. Raise your eyebrows as high as you can and then release them. Next, shut your eyes tightly and then release. Move on to your mouth and open it wide and stretch your jaw, now relax, and let your tongue hang for a moment. Continue with your neck by raising your shoulders to your ears and lowering them. Move along and tense and release your stomach and then your buttocks muscles. Continue to your arms and hands by squeezing your fingers into fists and then releasing. Continue to your legs and end by curling your toes forward and then releasing. As you tense each body part, inhale through your nose and hold the breath, and as you exhale, release the muscle. If you are really short on time, try to just practice the relaxation portion of the exercise on each muscle group. In addition to helping me to relax and fall asleep, I find this exercise very helpful when trying to manage my anxiety. You can play some soothing music while you do it.

Ask yourself the following:

- Do I keep a consistent sleep schedule, even on the weekends?

- Do I have established healthy, relaxing bedtime rituals? (I loved when Dr. Naiman warned that a ritual like Sleepy Time Tea could have the potential to lead to Pee-Pee Time Tea, so choose your rituals carefully!)

- Do I unplug at least an hour before bed? Do I have a proper sleep environment?

Your bedroom environment should be your sanctuary. It should be calming and relaxing, not cluttered with distractions that do not let you unwind. It should be very dark and cool. Pay attention to the type of conversations you have in your bedroom and try not to have important emotional conversations in your bedroom. Save those conversations for another room so that your bedroom is free from stress and negative energy. Make sure you have a good quality supportive mattress and bed linens that feel good on your skin. I often suggest that my clients use natural lotions before bed that contain lavender essential oils because the scent from these oils has a soothing effect on the mind and can help them to fall asleep.

Harmonious Tip:

Take a look around your bedroom. What is one simple thing you can do right now to improve the space to make it more conducive to help you catch some zzzzz's? Hormones that trigger hunger and satiety are released in our bodies and properly balanced when we have a good night's sleep. This leads us to make better, healthier food choices the next day, which leads to less physical discomfort and ultimately, less stress and fewer health problems. So be sure to get adequate amounts of sleep in a calm bedroom because the extra time you invest in sleeping will pay you back in greater productivity the next day.

BRING THE OUTDOORS INSIDE

Whenever you can, pause for a moment and open some windows in your home, and as the song says, "Let the sun shine in." It takes no time at all to crack open the windows, get some fresh air and help relieve the Nature Deficit Disorder so many of us suffer from. When you don't have time to get outside and spend time in nature, opening the windows is a quick and simple thing to do. It is very important for your detoxification system to breathe in fresh air, so air out your home. There are pollutants in the air we breathe in our homes caused by manmade chemicals. There are toxic substances in paints, building materials, the carpet in our homes, cleaning supplies, as well as on our clothing from our dry cleaning. These toxins can build up and be absorbed through our lungs if we do not air our homes out by opening the windows now and then. Removing toxic fumes from your home will reduce the number of headaches you experience, improve the air quality of your home, improve your mood, and improve your productivity.

No time to travel to paradise? Create a mini paradise filled with hints of nature in your home. Keeping plants in your home will not only make your indoor environment more beautiful, but it will also bring you physical and mental benefits.

Indoor plants help fight indoor pollutants and improve the air quality in your home. They also increase the humidity in the air which helps to prevent sore throats, coughs, and fatigue.

Being surrounded by plants, just like being in nature, can help improve your concentration, memory, and productivity. What I love most about having plants in my home is that it is a way of bringing the outdoors inside. Being in nature has a wonderful effect on our mood and bringing elements of nature indoors helps us recreate this effect in our homes.

Having plants forces you to focus your attention away from yourself and toward nurturing something else. As you water your plant, it feels great to know you are providing it with the nutrients it needs to thrive and grow. As you move your plants toward the sunlight, you connect with the benefit of sunlight. I have noticed that after I water my plants, I am often reminded to drink a glass of water and hydrate myself as well.

Some good plants to try to include are chrysanthemums, palms, peace lilies, snake plants, dieffenbachias, and bamboo palms. Do not be afraid to give this a try. You can start with a smaller sized plant and work your way up to a larger plant. I have definitely found a connection between taking care of my plants and my motivation to live a healthier and more relaxed lifestyle. Give it a try and see if nurturing your plants helps you remember to nurture yourself.

Harmonious Tip:

Set a time this week to go to a plant store and purchase a small plant, even a cactus will do, in a decorative holder that makes you smile. Notice it throughout the week, and spend a few minutes each day admiring it and watering it or pulling off the dry leaves. Notice how this small act has a positive effect on your stress by forcing you to slow down for a moment and connect with this tiny, lovely piece of nature. Your day won't be thrown off schedule if you devote a few minutes to this small piece of nature and appreciate it. Give it a try and you might discover you actually have a green thumb

Weather permitting, when you get home tomorrow evening, open the window in your bedroom, look outside for a moment, and inhale a long deep breath and then exhale. You will notice you feel much calmer and more relaxed when you open some windows and breathe in and smell the fresh air.

CHANGE YOUR TUNE

A simple, inexpensive, and effective tool that can shift your mood in your home immediately is listening to music.

Many ancient civilizations used music as a healing medium to affect their health and behavior. Today, music therapy helps individuals struggling with emotional, cognitive, and social issues because playing or listening to music helps them to express themselves. The healing benefits of music, however, can be enjoyed by anyone.

Listening to music can improve your mental wellbeing, and can boost your physical health. Valerie Salimpoor, a neuroscientist at McGill University in Montreal, observed PET scans of music lovers that showed large amounts of dopamine were released by their brains when the participants listened to music. Increased dopamine levels can make you happier. Listening to music at home can heighten your positive emotions by quieting your negative thoughts. This can distract you from the fear and negativity of negative thoughts, and help shift your mood. Having a heightened level of positive emotions is much better for your health and can even strengthen your immune system.

Just like the food we choose for our bodies is a very bio-individual choice, so is the type of music we choose to enjoy. The music that is right for you can fluctuate based on your activity, mood, and what your mind and body need at a particular point in time, in the same way that your food choices can change based upon your particular needs at a particular point in time. It is important to observe your body's response to various types of music to learn what is the best choice for you. Music choices are very subjective, and while slow music can relax us, some people find it depressing and it can actually cause them discomfort. Strong rhythmic music can affect your cardiovascular system by increasing your heart rate and breathing. It might be useful to listen to it at home when there is a task you need to perform because it will motivate you to move and keep alert. Softer music can help relax you, and classical music with complex patterns can help you draw on memories and neurological patterns that can help improve your brain health.

Harmonious Tip:

While it is great to turn on music in your home environment to help shift your mood or help you focus, don't forget to take your music with you. Listening to music in your car, on your commute, or even at work when possible can help release tension during the day and elevate your spirit. Playing soothing music before bed once you are back home will help you unwind, quiet your mind, and help you to sleep better as well.

CLEAR UP THE CLUTTER, BEAT THE CLOCK

Growing up, my sister and I shared a bedroom, and it was easy to tell which side was hers and which side was mine. Truth be told, as my family and husband will tell you, I am messy. However, since becoming a health coach, I have seen firsthand the connection between clutter and health, and have made great progress in decluttering.

I have visited clients who have the most gorgeous kitchens with granite counters perfectly suited for cooking, but they become too overwhelmed by their clutter to cook. When they clear out their drawers, they throw away or donate multiple spatulas, graters, and gadgets that they do not really need or use. When they pare down to just the basics so they can open their drawers and cabinets more easily, they are much more motivated to get into the kitchen and start cooking.

I often find the kitchen is a great place to begin to declutter. Go through your pantry. That hot chocolate mix that was in a holiday basket you received four years ago, that is probably loaded with chemicals, is expired, and can be tossed. Check expiration dates and toss anything that has expired. Read ingredient labels and throw out items that you know you will not use or should probably not be eating because it contains unhealthy chemicals. It is upsetting when we get rid of items we paid money for, but think about the health benefits.

I have a friend whose refrigerator is so organized she actually alphabetizes her yogurts and has them all facing forward so you can see the picture and the flavor. While I used to tease her about this, this strategy is actually brilliant. Having an organized refrigerator and pantry keeps you motivated to cook because finding ingredients when you are pressed for time is easy. I have found that storing seeds, nuts, grains, and beans in clear glass mason jars in my pantry is a great way to keep it neat, and allows me to easily grab what I need when I am cooking.

Once you have your kitchen decluttered and you feel motivated to cook more, you will be inspired to declutter the other rooms in your home. An organized bedroom closet is another area that can help you with your health. Why your bedroom closet? If you are rushed and stressed in the morning, rummaging through your closet trying to find pants that fit or the right belt or sweater, you will find yourself running late and likely might decide to skip breakfast or to not to pack your snacks. Having an organized closet will not only have a calming effect on your morning, but can help you regulate your eating.

Set a master plan and conquer spaces one small step at a time. Clearing clutter provides positive motivation in other areas of your health, not just in your food choices. Most notably, not looking at the clutter will immediately take a lot of stress off your mind because you are not constantly being reminded of things you have not dealt with or should be doing.

Harmonious Tip:

Find a friend, family member, or invest in a professional organizer. There is no shame in asking for help to declutter. Sometimes we are too attached to our possessions and we need a friend or family member to help us understand the costs versus benefits of holding on to certain items. Once you have chosen the items you are willing to part with, thank them for serving you, and if they can be donated, feel good about the joy they will bring to someone else. This act of letting go and helping others will have a huge impact on helping you create a calm and peaceful state of mind, and will save you tons of time searching for misplaced items amidst your clutter.

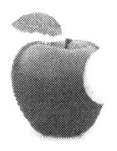

2
Healthy Eating

"One cannot think well, love well, or sleep well if one has not dined well."

- Virginia Woolf

Dining well does not have to mean eating in a five-star restaurant. It does not mean you have to invest large amounts of time and money. It means being aware of what you are putting into your body and the manner in which you eat it. You can prepare a lovely, simple, inexpensive pot of homemade soup filled with healthy vegetables, beans, and a grain, and sit around your kitchen table with your loved ones creating beautiful memories, sharing stories, and building relationships. You can also go to a five-star restaurant and be annoyed with the service, argue with your dinner companion, eat in a hurry without appreciating your food, and leave feeling upset that you wasted time, spent too much money, and now find yourself unable to unwind and relax.

Dining well means eating mindfully, chewing your food, drinking water before your meals, and eating with the seasons. Mindful eating does not take hours of time. It takes an awareness to appreciate your food and those you are sharing your meal with. Chewing your food longer might extend your meal time a bit, but the fact that it improves your digestive process will save you time later when that food exits your body in a more efficient manner! Drinking water throughout the day helps your body to eliminate toxins, and right now, as I am typing this, I quickly pause to take a sip of my water bottle, and I am back to typing in no time at all. (Just have a spill proof bottle so it doesn't spill on your laptop!) Eating with the seasons, my favorite tip of all for dining well, helps take the mystery out of what to eat, what to shop for, and will save you tons of time at the grocery store deciding what to purchase! Read on and see how just a little extra focus in adjusting your eating habits will save you lots of time wasted on digestive distress and trips to the doctor.

EAT MINDFULLY

To help manage cravings, prevent overeating, or eating too quickly, or to break away from conditioned habits of eating the wrong foods, learn to eat mindfully. Eating mindfully means becoming more conscious or aware of what and how you are eating. Doing this will greatly improve your eating habits as well as keep you more satisfied after a meal. Eating mindfully does not require additional time. It just requires different thought patterns while you are eating, and it has huge payoffs. It will help to ease any digestive problems you have, lessen your need to snack in the afternoon and evening, and give you better energy during the day to keep you more productive. You will notice your food tastes better and you enjoy it more when you eat mindfully. Here are some tips you can try one at a time to learn to eat mindfully.

- Pay attention to your hunger. If you are not sure if you are hungry, distract yourself, call a friend, drink some water, do some stretching, and then see if you are still truly hungry. We often look to food when we feel stressed but are not actually hungry. Noticing your hunger level is an important first step to take toward being a mindful eater, and to help eliminate emotional eating.

- Make sure you are eating your meals while seated and in a calm environment where you are not distracted or tense. Your eating environment should be pleasing, with everyone at the table in a relaxed state, not arguing or shouting. We take in not just the nutrients in our food, but also the energy around us during our mealtimes, so it is important that this energy is positive and nurturing.

- Try to only eat half of your plate, then sit for a minute or two, drink some water, and decide if you are truly hungry for more. If you still feel hungry, continue eating until you feel about 75% full. It takes some time for your brain to get the message that your stomach is full, therefore, it is important not to eat until you are stuffed, but to leave some room to allow for your brain to receive the signal that you are full.

- Try to visualize the farmer who grew your food and give appreciation to all the effort that went into getting it on your plate. Paying attention to the source and ingredients in your food is what making mindful choices and eating mindfully means. If there is a TV commercial for your food or you cannot pronounce items on its ingredients label, you probably should not eat it. If you are eating processed foods, it is often difficult to imagine the source from which it grew. Your food tastes better and you enjoy it more when you eat mindfully and when you stop using processed junk food to unwind and begin appreciating real whole food.

- Try to slow down when you eat, put your fork down between bites, and try to put less on the fork each time. Slowing down will improve your digestion and help prevent overeating.

I replaced my rushed lunch, which I often ate staring into my computer screen, and consisted of a salad where I tried to eat as little of the protein it was topped with for "fear" of gaining weight, with an appetizer that consisted of a short walk outside in the sun to unwind and soak up some Vitamin D. This allowed me time to bring about the relaxation response in my body so that when I ate lunch, I could do so mindfully and I digested it better. I gained back the time I used to go on the seven-minute walk at about 2:00pm when I no longer had gas pains from scoffing down my salad in a tense state and had to waste time in the ladies' room! After my walk, I ate a hearty, veggie packed meal topped with healthy protein and good fats with the new knowledge that the protein would keep my energy levels up and lasting later into the day, and the healthy fats, like avocado, would keep me more satisfied so I would not be tempted around 3:30pm to sabotage my efforts with M&M's or other junk that came across my line of vision. I carefully chewed my food, eating in a relaxed state, sitting quietly, away from my desk, appreciating the moment and my food. It was amazing how much more productive and effective I was completing tasks by spending more time eating in an empowered way with greater awareness.

Harmonious Tip:

Starting tomorrow morning with your breakfast, before you begin to eat, think about how you feel and look at your plate. Can you picture the food growing? Did it come from a plant in the ground, a tree, an animal? Take a deep breath and be thankful for the food you are about to consume. Before you stand up, breathe in and out twice, and notice how you feel differently from before you began eating. Mindful eating breaks the pace of your day, helps you regain composure and perspective, and renews you. Try this for a week and notice how much your body and mind start to shift to a calmer state.

DON'T BITE OFF MORE THAN YOU CAN CHEW

Many busy people tend to eat very quickly. They tend to get into the habit of rushing while they are eating, thinking about all the things they need to accomplish. When I teach my busy clients to eat mindfully, they stop thinking about how busy they are and instead start to focus on their food. Another way to help focus on your food is by chewing your food well.

"Why do I need to focus on my food?" asks the busy person. "I am only eating because I have to." My reply, "Why should you stop and smell the roses? Because single-minded focus helps you to become aware of the present moment, and become more grateful, which leads to greater happiness and ultimately greater health."

When you take time in the middle of the day to focus on your lunch and chew it well, you break the stress cycle you might have been in, and you return later with improved energy and focus.

Digestion begins in the mouth. As you start to chew your food, digestive enzymes found in saliva start to break down the food and prepare it for nutrient absorption. In order to get the most efficient absorption of minerals and vitamins, it is very important to thoroughly chew your food.

Pay attention to how much you are chewing your food, try to chew a little longer than usual, and really focus on the taste and flavor of your food. I often give clients a raisin and ask them to see how many times they can chew the raisin before they swallow it. Give this exercise a try. It will help you to notice your chewing habits and how to adjust them so that you are fully chewing your food for maximum absorption benefit and enjoyment.

If you are eating in a stressed state, standing, or rushing, it is likely that your saliva will be acidic. When you eat in a relaxed state, your saliva is more alkaline, and therefore, when you chew your food in a calm state, the food mixes with the saliva and your food becomes more alkaline. This allows the food to better absorb the acidic secretions in your stomach and can lead to less gas and less digestive distress.

When you do not chew your food properly, you leave large pieces of undigested food in your intestines where bacteria has to break it down. This can lead to gas, constipation, pain, and digestive problems. Your body releases digestive enzymes in the stomach when you chew and these enzymes break the food down and convert it to energy. So, the simple act of properly chewing your food can help you to avoid digestive distress and help your body gain more energy. Chewing slowly can also aid in weight loss because when you chew your food more thoroughly, you will become fuller and satisfied more quickly, and this will prevent you from overeating.

Some other tips to help you concentrate on chewing include taking smaller bites that will be easier to chew, and making sure your bite of food is thoroughly chewed and swallowed before taking another bite. While you are chewing, breathe deeply and concentrate on what you are doing. You will be surprised to see that when you adjust your chewing habits that your entire body will reap the benefits.

Harmonious Tip:

To get yourself to start chewing more, grab a raisin, almond, or other small nut or dried fruit and see how many times you can chew it before you need to swallow. Practice this for several weeks and concentrate on chewing more during your meals. You will notice as you chew more that you feel much more relaxed and satisfied when you consume a meal that is chewed well as opposed to one that you inhale quickly, leaving you feeling unsatisfied and uncomfortable. Your stomach and digestive system will thank you later for the extra time invested during the meal spent chewing. You will likely save time in the long run by having to make fewer trips to the restroom or your medicine cabinet. So, remember, don't bite off more than you can chew!

QUICK SWITCHES

If you are busy and constantly feeling challenged for time, you know how debilitating it is when you are experiencing uncomfortable symptoms of digestive distress such as bloating, gas, reflux, constipation, or any other aches or pains in your body. People often waste time and money going to the doctor for these symptoms, but it is a good idea to try to eliminate certain foods that are often associated with these symptoms for a short period of time to see if any of these symptoms are relieved or go away. The foods that I find most frequently cause people discomfort in their body, as well as with their mood and focus, are gluten, dairy, and sugar. I work with my clients to eliminate these foods from their diet for a few weeks, and then slowly introduce them back to see if they notice any changes. Often, they feel so great after they eliminate these foods they do not even want to add them back!

Rather than deprive yourself of certain foods, consider "crowding out" certain foods by adding in healthier options to your diet. Personally, I feel more energetic and have less brain fog and mood swings when I crowd these three ingredients out of my diet. Doing this also diminishes my cravings. Here are some strategies I have for crowding out each of these foods.

To crowd out dairy – Today's cows are fed hormones, antibiotics, and food that has been treated with pesticides, which all get into our milk supply and can cause potential risks to humans. But even without these added chemicals, it is unnatural for humans to be consuming cow's milk on a regular basis. Dairy can cause digestive problems for people with lactose intolerance and can aggravate irritable bowel syndrome. Personally, I feel much better experimenting with a variety of milk substitutes such as almond milk, rice milk, or coconut milk. Add in these alternative milks slowly. Start by using half regular milk and half alternative milk. After a few days, increase the percentage of alternative milk. Try experimenting with coconut or almond yogurts as well. For cheese substitutes, try using chopped nuts or nutritional yeast to toss on your food in place of cheese.

As I eliminated dairy, most notably cow's milk, from my morning routine, and switched it for some healthy almond milk in my morning smoothie made with frozen fruit, dark leafy greens, chia seeds, and just a few dates for sweetness in place of sugar, I could not believe how much better my concentration was until lunchtime.

To crowd out gluten – Gluten is a protein found in many grains. It is also found in all forms of wheat, barley, and rye, like in breads and pastas. It can also be found in unexpected foods like soy sauce, and it is hidden in most processed foods. As opposed to the protein found in meats, the protein in gluten can be very hard for the stomach to digest, and for people with celiac disease, it can make them very sick. Even if you do not have celiac disease, you can still develop a sensitivity to gluten. For some people, it can affect their joints, mood, or stomach, and can cause gas, fatigue, diarrhea, and mood swings.

As a health coach, people ask me all the time why were humans able to eat gluten for thousands of years with no problem but they can't eat it today? Thousands of years ago, when wheat was grown, it was stored, milled, and consumed, and it nourished mankind. Then, during the industrial age, machines would turn wheat into white flour. In an effort to yield crops faster, chemical and genetic technologies were developed by scientists to make the same wheat resistant to pests and droughts. All of this unnatural human intervention has made it more difficult in modern times for humans to digest gluten.

My old breakfast routine consisted of grabbing a quick, gluten filled cold cereal and a bowl of milk, or a bagel with some cream cheese that left me hungry and unsatisfied just an hour later. To kill the hunger pains, I would try to smother them with cups of hot coffee. This only served to raise my cortisol levels, making me more irritable, and consequently, without me knowing, making it even harder for me to lose those stubborn pounds that were making me unhappy and uncomfortable. This new smoothie routine, which didn't take very long to make once I developed a system, keeps me energized and motivated to drink more water before lunch to keep that focused feeling going in a healthy way. I've become so much more productive during the morning now and I aim to keep that energized feeling going as long as I can throughout the day.

Most of my clients who try crowding out gluten for a period of time find that they start to feel so much better that they never decide to add it back in. Everyone is different and some people can tolerate small amounts, but I would suggest that you try slowly crowding it out and see if you start to feel better. More and more gluten-free breads are showing up in health food stores. Brands such as Udi's make a large variety of breads, tortillas, and bagels that are gluten-free. There are also a lot of gluten-free corn chips and crackers in the stores. Keep in mind that while there are many gluten-free products in the stores, stocking up on these processed items is not necessarily a healthy choice. Even though these items do not contain gluten, many of them contain preservatives and other chemicals that are unhealthy. Read labels and use these products sparingly. When I first started to eliminate gluten, I often ate turkey sandwiches on large round brown rice cakes that I topped with mustard, lettuce, and tomatoes. I also tried wrapping my sandwiches in a piece of romaine lettuce or a large Swiss chard leaf, which was a delicious option. In place of pasta, I started incorporating more gluten-free grains into my diet such as brown rice and quinoa. Experiment with different recipes and you will find that it starts to become easier to crowd gluten out of your diet.

To crowd out sugar – Admittedly, crowding out sugar can be the most difficult for many people because humans naturally crave sugar. Even animals, as far back as apes millions of years ago, choose ripe fruit over unripe fruit because of its higher sugar content which gives them more energy. For all of you busy folks out there who are thinking about putting down my book right now because you are telling yourself, "Get rid of sugar? Yea, right, I have no time for that nonsense," please stay with me here. I will save you some time!

Refined, simple sugar which can go by the name sugar, cane sugar, brown sugar, corn syrup, high fructose corn syrup, or sucrose is absorbed into your body very quickly. Yes, that is great for the busy person who is low on energy and needs a fix fast! But here is how the cycle goes, and here is why eating refined sugar is actually the worst thing that the busy, time pressed person can do. Unlike eating complex carbs like fruits and vegetables, which release fiber into your blood, where your body processes the natural sugar slowly, simple sugar quickly raises your blood sugar levels. This causes the busy, stressed person to experience excitability and fills them with nervous tension, and can even cause hyperactivity. Not a good thing for you if you are busy and need to focus.

The body is an amazing machine and naturally wants to keep your blood sugar level steady, so the body secretes insulin to help lower the blood sugar level in the body after you bite into that candy bar. When your pancreas has to elevate its production of insulin, it reduces the production of a hormone called glucagon. (You are thinking, "I am busy and I want sugar. Why are you giving me a biology lesson?" but hang on!) You are busy, and you feel like you don't have time to go to the gym or to exercise, but maybe you want to lose weight or body fat? Well, glucagon production is very important for losing body fat because it allows stored body fat to be released into the blood stream and to be burned by your muscles as energy. So, if you are eating refined sugar like that candy bar, causing your pancreas to elevate its production of insulin while reducing its supply of glucagon, guess what you are actually doing. You are locking in excess body fat, making it even harder for your body to get rid of it.

Now, here you are, at your desk at work with a looming deadline, or rushing at the grocery store because you only have a few minutes until its carpool time, and suddenly, you are overwhelmed with an urgent sense of needing more fuel, more energy, more calories! The surge in insulin has lowered your blood sugar and now you are craving even more sugar because you need energy. You are circling around in this crazy sugar craving cycle like a hamster on a wheel, making no progress, and you are losing productivity and focus and wasting time.

I now find that when I do have real sugar, my taste buds are overly sensitive to it and I can't have much. Start by experimenting with a variety of natural sweeteners such as coconut nectar, raw honey, or maple syrup. Recipes that are sweetened with chopped dates or bananas are surprisingly satisfying. As your taste buds adjust to these new sweeteners, you will not miss the sugar. Another tip to help with the sugar cravings is to increase the amount of probiotics in your diet. By increasing the amount of healthy, good bacteria in your digestive system, you can destroy any yeast in your system, which is feeding off sugar and contributing to your cravings. There are probiotic drinks you can buy like kombucha, or you can even make your own sauerkraut, or you can take a probiotic in a capsule form. Increasing the amount of sea vegetables in your diet can help curb sugar cravings since sugar depletes the minerals in your body. Cook up some root vegetables to help curb your sugar cravings. As they cook they develop a sweet flavor that will satisfy you in a healthy way.

Harmonious Tip:

There are tons of recipes available on the internet that are gluten, dairy, and sugar-free. Don't be afraid to give these recipes a try. As you learn how to prepare them and experiment with new ingredients, you will find these recipes very satisfying and that they have a very positive impact on your health. If you eliminate these trigger foods and do not notice any changes or improvements, you can always just reintroduce them back into your diet later on. During this process though, you may find some new foods you actually enjoy. For those of you, like me, who find these foods are triggers for you, once you eliminate them from your diet and notice how wonderful you feel, you will be motivated and excited to continue adding new substitutes into your diet.

DRINK UP: KEEP YOUR HEAD ABOVE WATER

There are so many schools of thought about whether or not to drink water with your meals. Some say water with meals can have a negative impact on digestion by diluting digestive juices, while others say it acts as a lubricant and aids in digestion. I feel that the decision is a personal one and that people should experiment and see what works best for them. Personally, I find I need to sip just a bit of water during mealtimes, and have found that drinking room temperature water rather than ice water has a much better effect on my body when I drink during a meal. When we drink cold water, it may cause blood vessels in our stomach to shrink which slows digestion, so perhaps that is why I feel better when I drink room temperature water.

One thing is for sure and applies to everyone—staying hydrated throughout the day has a positive impact on your health. It improves digestion and regulates your mood. Drink eight 8-ounce glasses of water every day. As your body gets used to the additional water, you can adjust as needed. It is important to note that the amount of water you should drink during the day is a very individual matter and can vary based on the climate, altitude, and amount of exercise you do. If you are not drinking enough water during the day, you can become dehydrated which will lead to headaches or fatigue and a negative mood.

I recently started drinking a tall glass of water about thirty minutes before my meal and have noticed this helps me to feel better after the meal is over. I believe this is because drinking before the meal fills me up a little and then I tend not to overeat.

I also strongly recommend drinking a warm or room temperature cup of lemon water when you first wake up in the morning. The warm water is a great way to rehydrate your body after sleep, whereas cold water can shock your system when you first wake up. I find the warmth very soothing and comforting when I first wake up and ease into the day, and a little boost of Vitamin C in the morning is good for your adrenal glands and can give you an immune boost as well.

Harmonious Tip:

To motivate yourself to drink more throughout the day, get yourself a colorful glass or metal water bottle that you enjoy drinking out of, one that is pleasing to your eye or feels good in your hand. Keep it on your desk or in your bag as a reminder to stay hydrated during the day. As you increase your water intake, you will notice better skin, less cravings, and an overall increase in energy and mood.

EAT WITH THE SEASONS

Our ancestors ate seasonally because they had no choice. In spring and summer, when fresh greens grew and fruit ripened, that is what they consumed. In the fall, root vegetables made up a large part of the harvest, and in winter, people relied on animal food. Today, with highway transportation and refrigerated trucks, Americans can more or less eat whatever they want, anytime they want. However, learning to eat locally grown food according to the seasons will help you live more harmoniously with yourself, your body, and the earth.

Here are some simple ideas to try when trying to eat with the seasons. In winter, we naturally crave warming food. Foods that take longer to grow are generally more warming than foods that grow quickly. It is natural to crave animal food in winter because our bodies need to feel more solid and insulated from the cold. In winter, we should allow ourselves to eat heavier meals with plenty of oils, proteins, and nuts. If you are vegetarian, grilling your vegetables in the winter will give them more heat and density. You should save the raw vegetables and salads for summer and spring. Thick soups in winter, especially those with root vegetables including carrots, onions, and garlic will help keep your body feeling sturdy. In the summer, we love light foods from the farmer's market such as strawberries and fresh greens, so eating root vegetables that grow beneath the ground in summer can make us feel heavy.

I encourage you to begin to pay attention to eating seasonal food for the nutritional benefits. Seasonal foods are picked at the peak of freshness and offer higher nutritional content than out of season, unripe fruits and vegetables. Additionally, eating local foods helps protect our planet by reducing the number of miles your food has to travel before it reaches your plate. Also, local seasonal foods are priced much more economically than out of season foods and will save you money on your grocery bills.

I love cookbook author, Terry Walters, advice in her book, Clean Food: "Before you walk into a grocery store, a restaurant or even your own kitchen, pause, take a deep breath and connect with the intention to select only foods that will serve you." When you are in the supermarket making produce choices, choose vegetables and fruits grown in your local area which will ensure they are seasonal, and if possible, choose organic produce. Remember to check the frozen aisles for organic produce if there are no sustainable fruit or vegetable options in your supermarket. Frozen produce is a good option for a busy person who has an unpredictable schedule because your fresh produce will not go to waste if you suddenly are unable to use your produce during an unexpected busy week. When fresh local produce is not an option, I would always choose frozen over canned for its superior nutritional value.

Another simple way to eat locally and seasonally is to shop at farmer's markets if there is one in your area. Another great option is to join a Community Supported Agriculture (CSA), which helps farmers in need of income and busy families in need of fresh produce. For the very busy person who has trouble getting to the grocery store or the farmer's market, there are new companies springing up in some parts of the country that will keep you stocked with fresh vegetables and produce delivered from local farmers right to your home or office. Some of these companies will even deliver local pasture raised meat and eggs and other natural staples for your pantry. These companies partner with local farmers and ranchers to deliver high quality, sustainably produced, seasonal local food, which support your health and your community.

Harmonious Tip:

Think about one fruit and one vegetable that is in season right now, and on your next trip to the store, purchase some of each. Think about a recipe you might enjoy preparing with this food, or just bite into it and enjoy it raw. Think about the fact that you cannot find this tasting so fresh at other points in the year. Eating with the seasons helps us to become more aware of nature's cycles and is a natural way to help us vary our diet. By eating a varied diet, we are less likely to develop food intolerances. Becoming more aware of nature's cycles helps us develop a greater appreciation for our surroundings, our food, and makes us feel more balanced, grounded, happy, and secure.

FOOD AND FINANCES

As a former CPA turned health coach, I am interested in the relationship between our finances and our food choices, specifically how financial pressures around money impact our food choices, and some of the common misconceptions about the cost of healthy food versus unhealthy food.

When I left the corporate world and moved to Dallas to work with small business owners, I started to notice a pattern. The businesses that were in strong financial health typically seemed to have business owners who were in fairly good physical health. Not surprisingly, business owners who were disciplined about their eating habits and exercise were better capable of being disciplined concerning impulse buying, saving money on a consistent basis, and staying positive.

A 2014 study from the Olin Business School at Washington University in St. Louis found that retirement savings and health improvement behaviors are highly correlated. The study found that "those who save for the future by contributing to a 401(k) improved abnormal health test results and poor health behaviors approximately 27% more than non-contributors." (Schoenherr, Neil. Poor Physical, Financial Health Driven by Same Factors. The Source. Olin Business School. Washington University, St. Louis, 2014. Web.)

When people feel in control of their finances, their stress levels go down and that improves their attitude which typically improves their energy and focus, allowing them to be more productive at work. I have definitely found that financial wellness promotes healthier behaviors and attitudes in all areas of a person's life and this leads to happier and healthier feelings.

During my career as a CPA and now as a health coach, I have seen all the negative effects that financial pressure has on someone's health. Financial stress can be due to a job loss, medical bills, debt, or unexpected expenses. It can often lead to severe anxiety and depression, which of course, has a terrible effect on your body and health. Relationships tend to suffer when there is financial pressure. Financial pressure will effect appetite and sleep and very often impacts how regularly someone will go to see their doctor.

At some point or another, financial pressure will touch most people, and it is how they cope with the pressure as well as their ability to continue to invest in their health that determines how successful they'll be. Something I often hear from people is that "it's so expensive to eat healthy." I get so frustrated hearing this because my own analysis has proved the opposite.

There are a lot of misconceptions about the cost of healthy food. I have heard from so many people that healthy food is so much more expensive than unhealthy food. I think a lot of people are leery of shopping at places like Whole Foods because of this attitude. If someone is feeling financial pressure and has this attitude, they certainly will not be interested in healthy eating. To some degree it is true that healthy food sometimes costs more, take for example, an organic free-range, grass-fed piece of meat versus a brand name package of that same cut of meat. However, I have found several examples where healthier food choices actually cost less.

Often, I see boxes of grains in my client's pantries that include a spice packet. These boxes are much more expensive than purchasing grains from the bulk section of the grocery store and then using spices and herbs to season the grains. In addition to the cost savings, generally these boxes with spice packets contain added chemicals and preservatives that are bad for our digestion. Another client I had was spending money on individual containers of yogurt. I had her buy a few glass mason jars, and showed her a simple way to mix a large container of plain yogurt with frozen fruit, some chia seeds, and some cinnamon into portions and put that into the mason jars. She said it took her under fifteen minutes to prepare, and she liked them better. Plus, adding in the chia seeds kept her full longer so she was snacking less which saved money as well. She saved a lot of money by reusing the mason jars each week, not to mention, eliminating the almost six teaspoons of sugar that were hidden in her individual portion yogurt containers. Another benefit of the mason jars is that they are better for the environment.

When I work with clients to teach them to eat healthier, they are often surprised when they see that their grocery bills are lower. This makes the investment in a health coach well worth it because chances are you will recover the investment and even save money on medications, doctor's visits, processed food choices, unnecessary diet powders and supplements, and less missed days from work. Saving money and eating healthier is a great combination. As Gandhi said, "It is health that is real wealth and not pieces of gold and silver."

I find that as people become more stressed about their finances, they lose their ability to stay focused on the tasks involved with meal planning. This is one of the areas where I find the most satisfaction in helping others. When I am able to redirect that stress into focusing on cooking and meal planning with the goal of not just maintaining health but also saving money, clients start to feel better, work more effectively, or have more focus and energy to look for a better job, or to improve their current situation.

Just as taking care of one's health is an ongoing journey, so is taking care of one's finances. Just like we must be disciplined each week to invest in our health with proper nutrition and diet, we must continue to invest in and assess our portfolios on a regular basis, making changes when necessary, just as we do with our nutrition and lifestyle choices. Discipline and focus is necessary to maintain good physical and financial health habits.

Harmonious Tip:

Are you feeling pressure about your current or future financial circumstances? If so, consider focusing on your financial health by working with an advisor who can continuously review your financial situation with you and make suggestions. When you have a clearer understanding of your finances, this will lead to less stress and worry and less health related problems. It will also save you a lot of wasted time spent worrying about things, and instead, allow you to take action.

3

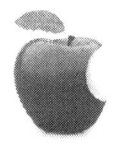

Healthy Body

*"Take care of your body.
It's the only place you have to live."*

- Jim Rohn

In my religion, the Jewish understanding of the body is that the body was created in the image of God. According to the Christian religion, the apostle, Paul, says your body is a temple of the Holy Spirit who is in you, whom you have received from God. He teaches that you should honor God with your body. And according to Hindu scriptures, the human body is the temple of God.

Ancient religions understood the value and importance of our human bodies, yet in modern day, many people take better care of their cars than they do their bodies. Often, it seems people only stop to think about the health of their bodies when something is wrong. Honoring our bodies and taking care of them every day, treating them with respect is crucial if we hope to maintain good health and live a happy, productive, long life. In this chapter, I provide some simple tips to care for your body such as dry skin brushing, using a tongue cleaner, movement, using safe personal care products, and stress management techniques. While the dry skin brush will undoubtedly add some extra time to your morning routine, the added energy you will feel from increased circulation can save you time at Starbucks, at the coffee pot in the office, or at the soda machine. For the price of about three cups of Starbucks, you can own a dry skin brush that can last for years. Using a tongue cleaner takes about a minute and will help minimize food cravings. Just think how much time you spend thinking about, fighting, or giving in to mid-day cravings. Surely that is more than a minute. Adding forms of movement into your daily routine to keep your body functioning at its peak capacity does not have to take up hours of your time in a gym, and when you are able to identify the proper type of movement that works for your body, you will be motivated to keep with it. A simple switch and awareness of ingredients in your personal care products can help your body look and feel its best. Finally, incorporating some stress management techniques into your daily routine will help bring about a relaxed state in your body, and allow it to better handle the toxins it encounters on a daily basis, leading to less illness.

BRUSH YOUR SKIN

Your skin is your largest organ and adding dry skin brushing into your daily routine can provide many health benefits. Dry skin brushing is good for your lymphatic system which is responsible for eliminating toxins and waste from your body. Toxins can build up and make you sick when your lymphatic system is not working, so it is important to stimulate it to help it release toxins, and dry skin brushing provides that stimulation. Dry skin brushing also helps to exfoliate your skin which will help to unclog pores and keep your skin looking healthy by removing dead skin.

To start, look for a high quality skin brush that has natural bristles and one with a long handle for hard to reach spots. An average dry skin brushing session can last anywhere from one minute to ten minutes, and for the best results, should be done daily. I prefer to do mine before my morning shower.

When using the dry skin brush, always brush toward your heart to promote circulation and lymphatic drainage. You can brush your entire body including your legs, arms, chest, back, stomach, and the bottoms of your feet. Avoid your face and other delicate areas. The pressure should not be painful, but should be firm enough so that you feel invigorated. Your skin may be a little pink after the session as blood starts circulating to the outer layers of your skin, but should not be irritated.

After the dry skin massage, it is good to rinse off in the shower.

After the shower, massage your skin dry with a towel, and then rub some natural oil, such as almond, coconut, or jojoba into the skin to keep it moisturized.

Harmonious Tip:

Check your natural grocery store or online for a natural dry skin brush. You can usually find them for under $20. This is an easy way to bring you more in touch with your body while exfoliating your skin and eliminating toxins to help you look and feel your best.

DITCH YOUR ALL-OR-NOTHING ATTITUDE

As far as exercise is concerned (or movement, as I prefer to call it), I have always fallen into the all-or-nothing category. If I was not in the mood for a full workout, whether it be an exercise class, a yoga class, a workout video, a full three mile run, or my twenty-five minutes on a machine at the gym, then my default strategy was to do nothing.

Maybe these excuses sound familiar to you: Well, if I can't get motivated to go running, what good will a walk around the block do? I have so much to do in the house anyway! If I will not make it to the exercise class on time, what is the point of just going to the gym to use the machines and walk on the treadmill? I should do laundry instead. If I can't make it to yoga class, how helpful would it really be if I just do a couple of yoga poses for five minutes? I'll catch up on Facebook instead.

The thing is, a short walk around the block will do a ton of good. It will clear your head, give you a change of scenery, relax your mood, and possibly even motivate you to actually go for a run. Parking far away from the store or the office, or forcing yourself to use the stairs instead of the elevator will give you a boost of energy and the positive feeling that you are being proactive, which will boost your self-confidence. Starting your morning by doing a few simple yoga poses and stretches can have lasting effects on your entire day, can remind you to keep your shoulders relaxed, prevent headaches later in the day, and can release any stress you might not even realize you are carrying in your body.

Ever since I have eliminated the all-or-nothing approach, I have been happily surprised at how the simplest form of movement—a walk in the neighborhood, some stretches on my mat, or even just some quiet time seated, taking some deep breaths—can actually have a profound effect on my mood and my body for the day. The biggest benefit I have found is how I feel about myself. I no longer hear negative self-talk like, "You are so lazy, you skipped the gym today," or, "You are going to regret not using the treadmill today next time you try to go for a run," or, "You really should have used the exercise DVD this morning. Now you are going to feel out of shape." Instead, I feel proud of myself and think, "That was a great walk today. You got fresh air and did some quiet thinking over an issue you needed to resolve," or, "My shoulder feels so much better. I am so glad I stretched this morning. I should do that again tonight," or, "I can't believe I didn't get angry over the phone call I just had. I bet the breathing and quiet time I had this morning helped me."

If you are a busy person and you do not have a lot of free time in your day for a full workout, it is important to understand that squeezing in any movement during the course of your day will actually add up over the course of a week, and will positively affect your health. It is important to understand that the type of movement that you choose is the right choice for your body, your schedule, and your mind. Just like food is very bio-individual and not all types of dietary plans are right for all people, not all forms of exercise are right for everyone. As I mentioned in my introduction, it is very important that the movement you choose for your body and personality resonates with you, because if not, it will be very hard for you to make it a habit. When I was trying to force myself to go to that loud aerobics class at my gym, I could not stay motivated to do it. When I understood that what I needed in the morning was gentle, flowing stretches to wake up my body slowly and calmly, I was better able to stick with it on a more consistent basis.

Harmonious Tip:

Releasing the all-or-nothing approach gives us permission to do what we can on some days, and appreciate an awesome workout on days when we can give it our all. Every time we take even the smallest step forward toward moving our body, we are providing our body and mind with huge health benefits. Being at peace with our exercise routine, feeling positive toward what we did for our body rather than guilt is a gift for your mind as well as your body. Appreciate every form of movement your amazing body can do. Remember this quote by Edward Stanley: "Those who think they have no time for bodily exercise will sooner or later have to find time for illness."

GIVE YOUR STOMACH ACID A BOOST

Acid in your stomach helps to kill any viruses and bacteria you might ingest, and also helps the food in your stomach to digest quickly instead of refluxing backward into your esophagus. Stomach acid also helps to activate digestive enzymes which help digest protein properly for a healthy immune system, as well as helps our bodies absorb important nutrients.

Signs of low stomach acid include heartburn, belching or gas, bloating, fatigue, headaches, diarrhea, indigestion, and nausea. Some health conditions associated with low stomach acid include allergies, asthma, autoimmune disease, dry skin, eczema, and chronic fatigue syndrome.

When you have prolonged periods of time where your schedule is very busy or you are under unusual amounts of stress, a negative impact on your digestive system is created because stress slows down the digestive system and activates your fight or flight response. Think back to the days when our ancestors were hunting for food, and perhaps suddenly encountered a dangerous threat such as an animal approaching them, about to attack. The hunter becomes stressed, and the human body, being the amazing machine that it is, knows exactly what to do in this situation. The central nervous system shut down blood flow to the digestive system, slowing the contractions of digestive muscles and the secretions needed for digestion. Instead, blood flow was redirected to the brain and muscles, which allowed our ancestors to better fight or run away (flight).

While that response was fine for our ancestor hunters, it is not fine for modern day, busy, stressed people.

When our ancestors spent time hunting, the fight or flight response was triggered by the sympathetic nervous system, and that activated a response in the body which caused rapid breathing and the heart to race. It also stimulated the release of cortisol, which kept their blood sugar levels elevated so they would have energy to run. Then, after the hunt was over, our ancestor hunter went back to his hut or his cave, and guess what he did. He rested from that hard fight. As he rested, his hormone levels returned to normal, and his blood sugar went back down, and blood flow returned to his digestive system. After he rested, as he ate his recent conquest, his body was in perfect condition to properly digest his prey. He did not need any tums.

Modern day people are living in a constant state of stress, running from activity to activity, and not allowing their bodies to return to a proper state of rest to digest their food. The argument with your client, the email on your device, the text from your boss or child, it is constant, and your body thinks a big giant bear is after you all the time. Many of us are living in a constant state of fight or flight, and our bodies are not wired for digesting food because our brains think the body must preserve all of its energy to handle a potential threat.

Many people mistakenly think that some of the symptoms of low stomach acid are caused by having too much acid in their system, and they take acid blocking drugs which come with health risks such as osteoporosis and kidney damage.

A more natural and safer solution is to boost your stomach acid by adding a small amount of fresh lemon juice or fermented apple cider vinegar to warm or room temperature water about twenty minutes before you eat. This increases the production of hydrochloric acid in your body, which aids in protein digestion and kills bacteria that can enter the body through food.

Here are some other things you can do to break out of the fight or flight response and allow your body the responses it needs to properly digest your food, so you do not experience digestive pain, heartburn, and reflux, and allow your stomach acid secretions to remain in balance.

- Take time to relax your body when you eat by eating in a calm, relaxed state, sitting down, and chewing your food thoroughly.

- Try eating smaller meals throughout the day. Sometimes larger meals can put strain on the lower esophageal sphincter (the sphincter that closes the esophagus from the stomach), causing it to spasm. This allows stomach acid to enter the esophagus and causes irritation and pain.

- Drink less liquids with your meals so you don't dilute stomach acid.

Remember we are all individual, some of these tips will work for you and your lifestyle and perhaps some will not, so experiment to see which help you feel better and eliminate digestive discomfort.

Personally, I have noticed that when I incorporate the ritual of drinking warm lemon water or apple cider vinegar on an empty stomach before breakfast, not only is my digestion greatly improved, I experience fewer cravings throughout the day, and my energy level is more consistent. Give it a try and see how you feel. If the taste is hard to get used to, you can add a small amount of honey to the mixture until you get used to it. I enjoy drinking it in a mug with warm water as I find the warmth comforting and I love knowing I am doing something good for my body. Experiment with a water mixture—a combination of lemon juice, apple cider vinegar, and honey with a dash of ginger is a great, natural digestive aid for your body. I have even gotten to the point of enjoying the tangy taste of the apple cider vinegar in my water alone.

Harmonious Tip:

Eating fermented foods is another way to increase your stomach acid while adding beneficial bacteria to your digestive system. Thinly slice up a head of cabbage, massage it in a large bowl with a tablespoon of a good quality sea salt until it becomes limp and releases its juice. Store in in a sealed, air tight container for a few weeks, then transfer to the refrigerator. Eat a small portion with your meals including the juice. Sauerkraut and cabbage juice are strong stimulants for your body to produce stomach acid, which will do wonders for your digestion. Better digestion means less stress on your body, which means a happier, more energetic you!

HEALTH FOR THE TIP OF YOUR TONGUE

My dentist never told me about tongue cleaners. I learned about them in nutrition school. Tongue cleaners originated thousands of years ago as an Ayurvedic self-care ritual to remove toxic debris from the tongue's surface. According to Ayurveda, a tongue that is clean and clear of debris indicates a clear mind and body.

Today, tongue cleaners can be used to clean bacterial buildup and food particles from the surface of the tongue. By removing bacteria from the tongue, we can minimize oral care problems such as halitosis (bad breath). There is a link between oral health and systemic disease in the rest of the body, so maximizing your oral health is good for the rest of your body as well. Our mouths contain bacteria and these bacteria can disseminate to other parts of the body. Infections in the mouth can lead to disease in the body. In fact, gum infections can cause other health conditions with some research indicating it may be associated with heart disease, diabetes, or stroke.

By cleaning food bacteria off the tongue, your taste buds can more fully experience subtle flavors in your food. This leads to greater mealtime satisfaction, and can lead to less snacking because you do not need as much added salt and sugar when your mealtime food tastes better and leaves you more satisfied. I have also noticed when using the tongue cleaner myself that when food particles remain on my tongue (especially after a heavy meat meal), I find myself craving sweets. When I use the tongue cleaner after a meal, I find it helps reduce my cravings. My clients have noted that they feel similar effects and that they love the feeling of freshness in their mouth after using the tongue cleaner.

Use the round edge of the tongue cleaner and gently scrape down on your tongue with mild pressure. Do this two or three times, making sure not to go too far back into your mouth. You do not want to choke or scrape the salivary glands at the back of your tongue. Rinse the scraper under water and repeat until your tongue is clear.

There are many different tongue scrapers on the market today, but the one I enjoy is a soft copper metal U-shape. I suggest avoiding any tongue cleaners that have bristles because I find these serve to move the bacteria around, but are not as effective at removing it. You can use the tongue scraper at home after you brush your teeth in the evening. Also, consider keeping a tongue scraper in your purse or bag so it is easily accessible and can be used after lunch to clear your tongue of any leftover food particles, to eliminate bacteria, and to help reduce afternoon cravings. The tongue scraper can also reduce excess mucus, and in turn, clear up any congestion in your nose or throat.

Harmonious Tip:

Find a copper U-shaped tongue cleaner and give it a try. By cleaning your tongue, you begin to pay attention to the coating on your tongue that may have built up from years of poor food choices or toxins resulting from poor digestion, and this can help motivate you to focus on making healthier choices. Notice how nice it is to have a fresh taste in your mouth, and how any after meal cravings you usually have begin to subside when you use the tongue cleaner. In addition, your fresh mouth will inspire you to kiss your honey more! This alone is a definite stress buster.

READ YOUR PERSONAL CARE PRODUCT LABELS

What you put on your skin ends up in your body. Because skin is semipermeable, it actually transports nutrients and other matter from its surface into the bloodstream and organs. Many of the personal care products that we use on our skin such as soap, body wash, deodorant, face creams, and shampoos contain chemicals that have been tested and proven to be endocrine disruptors. Endocrine disruptors are chemicals that, in certain doses, can interfere with the hormone system in mammals. These disruptions can lead to cancerous tumors, reproductive problems, developmental disorders, and allergies.

Fragrances found in many personal care products are made using petroleum or coal and can cause skin irritation as well as harm the environment. Fragrances made with cheap synthetic chemicals are used to replace the natural scents that come from elements already existing in nature. Organic essential oils are liquids that are distilled (most frequently by steam or water) from the leaves, stems, flowers, bark, roots, or other elements of a plant. The chemical composition and aroma of essential oils can provide valuable psychological and physical therapeutic benefits. It is cheaper for companies to use synthetic chemicals due to the higher price and limited availability of essential oils, which are natural.

Due to a loophole in the Federal Fair Packaging and Labeling Act, it is legal for companies not to list all the chemicals used in body care products on their labels. This is because companies purchase their fragrance mixtures from fragrance houses, who create the scents. Years ago, these companies lobbied to protect their secret fragrance formulas, and therefore, labels may just use the word "fragrance" or "parfum." Companies are not required to list all of the solvents, stabilizers, dyes, and preservatives contained in their products on their labels because trade secrets protect their privacy. They are also exempt from being listed by the U.S. Food & Drug Administration. Therefore, when you see the word "parfum," "perfume," or "fragrance" listed on your personal care products, you should be aware that these products may contain disrupting chemicals in them.

A simple way to begin is to swap your body moisturizer that may have irritants for a simple almond oil. Massage this into your skin after you shower and while it is drying, do some simple stretches. The stretches will loosen your muscles and increase circulation which will help keep you better energized throughout the day, and the added benefit of removing unnecessary and potentially dangerous chemicals and unnatural fragrances will not bog down your body, allowing it to be as productive as possible.

Look for products made by companies that use all natural ingredients and who fully disclose ingredient information on their packaging. I love using products from companies that use organic, natural, safe, plant based ingredients. Ever since I have switched to using these natural personal care products, I have noticed my skin is smoother, clearer, and less itchy, and my hair is fuller and less dry. If you can't pronounce the ingredients and it is full of preservatives and chemicals, search for more natural products.

Try swapping out your heavy fragrances and perfumes for other naturally scented essential oils. At your natural food grocer, you can often find roller balls filled with lovely smelling combinations of bergamot patchouli, ylang ylang, lavender, and other citrus oils. Try substituting these for your usual perfumes or try an all-natural spray.

Harmonious Tip:

Personal care products for our bodies filled with unnatural ingredients can get into our pores and into our bloodstream. As you make the switch to using more natural products, do not forget about your cleaning products and room deodorizers that also can get on your skin and into your lungs. Look for natural products free from harsh chemicals, and just like you should do with your food labels, read all of these labels and be sure you understand what the ingredients are. This will protect your physical health, and minimize discomfort in your body due to a lower toxic build-up. You will notice the more you use these natural products scented with essential oils, that they have an incredibly soothing effect on your mind and wellbeing.

WHO YA GONNA CALL? ...STRESS BUSTERS

Ninety percent of Americans think that stress contributes to illness, but only thirty percent think it has a direct impact on them. Stress affects all of us, and the problem with uncontrolled chronic stress is that it slowly attacks your body in ways you cannot always see. It is much later that signs of stress start to show themselves in your digestive tract, muscles, joints, sex hormones, skin, and hair.

Uncontrolled stress leads to inflammation in the body. Inflammation is the body's attempt to protect itself. It is a response by the body to try to remove anything it detects as being harmful or irritating.

Let's think about it in terms of a splinter. A strange piece of wood punctures your skin. Your immune system rushes to send help to that area to fight off any virus or toxin that may have gotten in. In an attempt to isolate that area from the rest of the body, your amazing immune system sends immune cells and molecules to the area that promote healing. That red, puffy swelling you see on your finger is inflammation, and that is good inflammation because it is acute. It is short lived. It signals the body to control the immune system, control infection, and to regrow damaged tissue.

Another type inflammation is called chronic inflammation, which is the inflammation I had in my body when I was doing a double shift, working, taking care of my family at a frantic pace, and not taking care of my health. It was really a combination of what Dr. Libby Weaver refers to as "chaos and comedy." I would scream at my kids or my husband and then get mad at myself. Dr. Weaver actually coined a phrase for this type of chronic stress that causes chronic inflammation—Rushing Women's Syndrome. Modern day women have their mother's responsibilities and their father's jobs, and they are exhausted. We want to be good enough, attractive enough, thin enough, smart enough, reply to emails fast enough, but enough is enough!!

I don't want to give you too much science here, but briefly, your adrenal glands are two little triangle shaped glands that sit above your kidneys and are responsible for your flight or fight response. In response to stress, they release Cortisol (adrenaline), which we need for survival. But if we are in a state of constant stress, these hormones can't turn off, and over time, it leads to a chronic inflammatory response in the body. Your body's immune system is constantly trying to fight the added chemicals in your system. Unlike the splinter, we often can't see this type of inflammation. The problem is that even though we cannot see it, it is there, and it is slowly damaging our bodies and leading to many diseases such as cancer, heart disease, asthma, Alzheimer's, and depression.

This chronic state of stress also creates adrenal fatigue, which makes it hard to lose weight. My clients are often delighted when I work with them on reducing stress and inflammation because they generally tend to lose several pounds as well.

It's important for people not to wait until chronic inflammation is detectable on the outside in the form of weight gain, dry and thinning hair, skin breakouts, digestive system bloating, constipation, gas, heartburn, or acid reflux. Poor food choices and sleep deprivation are common sources that contribute to chronic inflammatory stress and can become a health problem if they are constant. Working as a health coach, supporting my clients to make better food choices, and working with them on improving their sleep hygiene are often the first steps in reducing chronic inflammatory stress.

The next step is teaching clients how to nurture themselves. As a health coach, I often find myself in discussions with clients about the difference between what is self-care and what is selfish. Women especially find it difficult to take time out of their day, to do something that is dedicated to themselves, and often feel they are being selfish. The problem is that when we do not take time for ourselves, stress that could be temporary can turn into chronic stress, which as discussed above, leads to inflammation and all the health problems associated with it. We need to find a way to break the stress cycle and to tell our brains that everything is okay. Spend some time now developing a self-care practice so you do not have to spend time down the road dealing with an illness. You do not need to spend a lot of money on any of these self-care techniques.

Some examples include:

- Schedule a bubble bath for yourself one night a week,

and take time to soak in the tub with soothing music and a scented candle.

- Ride in silence in your car with no cell phone or radio and just be mindful of the view.

- Call a friend you have not spoken to in a while to chat and catch up.

- Indulge in high quality dark chocolate while you listen to music.

- Take a short walk after dinner.

- Spend some time in your garden.

Harmonious Tip:

The key to nurturing yourself is having support. In some cases, it's a friend or a spouse, and for many of my clients, it's me as their health coach. Find ways to manage psychological and social stress so it isn't preying on your mind. When you nurture yourself, you will find that you will be more productive while conveying to others that you value yourself, which will make you happier about your life. Treating yourself to something special can have an emotional and spiritual effect. It gives you the ability to be a better caregiver. When you nurture yourself, you trigger the relaxation response in your body, so in addition to less stress, the relaxation response boosts your immunity which leads to less illness. Another benefit many of my clients have noticed is that less stress leads to less emotional eating.

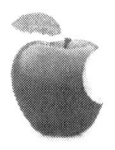

4
Healthy Cooking

"You don't have to cook fancy or complicated masterpieces, just good food from fresh ingredients."

- Julia Child

Julia Child did not grow up cooking, and I recently read that her mother rarely cooked. In fact, Julia did not learn to cook until she was thirty-two, proving that we can learn to cook well, even if we we're not exposed to cooking at a young age. Throughout history, many people avoided cooking and hoped to be able to hire others to do it for them. But let's face it, most of us cannot afford to hire chefs to cook for us full time in our homes, and learning to embrace the cooking process helps us to feel more connected to our bodies and to our food source. In Michael Pollan's book, *Cooked*, he urges us to start to value cooking, "It's the collapse of home cooking that led directly to the obesity epidemic." Our society has come to devalue cooking, and unfortunately, this is hurting our agriculture and our environment because we are letting large corporations do our cooking. When people stop cooking at home, they are not supporting diverse local farms, and they are inadvertently supporting large grain and animal factories. When we stop cooking at home, we stop connecting to the world around us.

My intent is to show you why it is worth investing a little time in the kitchen. We do not need to cook complex recipes. Keeping it simple will nourish us and make the cooking process more enjoyable. The energy, or prana, in our food is felt when food is prepared in a home with love and not by large industrial corporations, and this prana leads to better health. There is also a beautiful energy when a family sits around the dinner table together, sharing the same home cooked meal, as opposed to bringing in takeout food where each person is eating a different type of food prepared by a large corporation, and certainly a different energy if each person in the family is just individually nuking their microwaved meal. People underestimate how this beautiful energy affects them, their family, and how they actually end up wasting a lot of time searching for connections in other ways like through social media for example.

Personally, I found that as I began to cook more at home, I began to gain more energy, and that made me more excited to try new recipes and embrace the cooking process even more throughout my weekly routine. Cooking also got easier the more I did it, so I became more efficient at it and could prepare beautiful meals in less time. When I got home late in the evening from work or a kid's activity, and remembered that there was a huge, healthy pot of homemade turkey chili with beans and veggies in the refrigerator, I felt like I hit the jackpot. It only took a small amount of extra time on Sunday to plan ahead, swing by the grocery store to purchase the chili ingredients, chop up the veggies, and place them in the crockpot, but the benefit on a dark, cold evening, after a long, stressful day was amazing. I didn't have to eat a cold bowl of soggy cereal for dinner, or microwave some processed and unsatisfying frozen meal. Instead, I felt nourished and renewed by my advanced preparation. I was fueling my body with clean whole foods that left me with more energy and were much better for my digestion.

Learning to prep your food in advance will help minimize cooking time during the busy work week, and learning to use kitchen gadgets that make cooking simpler and more enjoyable will help the busy person navigate their way more easily around the kitchen. Experimenting with various spices and herbs will allow you to explore your creativity when cooking and will also make the process more fun, with the added benefit of aiding your digestion.

IS THERE PRANA IN YOUR FOOD?

Prana is a Sanskrit word that means life force. Prana gives us energy and can enter our bodies through food. Okay, don't roll your eyes and skip this section. Give it a chance! I also snubbed the concept at first, but it has actually really helped me enjoy preparing meals for my family. Okay, truth be told, I still may not enjoy cleaning the kitchen, but read on...

Prana exists in fresh foods, so think about food that is canned, frozen, old, microwaved, and processed as having less prana. Organic, local, and seasonal fruits and vegetables are very high in prana.

The most fascinating thing I discovered about prana through my own healing was that while we take in prana through the type of food we eat, the prana of our food is also affected by the mood of the cook who prepares it. Consider this quote by D.L Chopra, the father and mentor of Deepak Chopra: "*Prana is the vital life force of the universe...and it goes into you, into me, with food. When you cook with love, you transfer the love into the food and it is metabolized [when you eat]*." These beliefs are based on ancient Hindu scripture that encourages cooking food with love. I think about my childhood and eating my grandmother's chicken soup, and I am certain there was prana in that bowl.

Many religions have a similar concept that focuses on rituals around the preparation of food. My own religion, Judaism, has dietary laws which honor the sanctity of our food and encourages food preparation in an ethical and compassionate manner. Judaism provides strict regulations that instruct us on the limited types of animals we may consume as well as the methods of slaughter for permitted meats that lead to more humane killing of animals for human consumption. These methods are quick and less painful than today's corporate mass production meat and poultry industry methods.

To improve the nutritional value and the enjoyment of the food you prepare, it is important to focus on your mental state while preparing your food. We need to relax and calm down, and not feel like we are racing to get the meal on the table. I teach my clients to cook delicious and satisfying meals simply, in a short period of time, with confidence, ease, and a sense of happiness and appreciation. The mood of the cook definitely influences the quality of the food prepared. I have seen this in my own cooking, and I have heard this from many of my clients. When I come home from a long day, prepare a soothing cup of tea, change into comfortable clothing, turn on some music I love, and prepare simple food with just a few ingredients, my meals are beautiful, nurturing, and comforting. When I feel grateful and happy that I am preparing food for people I love, the cooking process is much more enjoyable and my food always comes out better. When I feel stressed and hurried, I often spill and burn my food and the quality is not the same.

When part of your meal is partially prepared in advance, it makes putting dinner together much quicker and simpler and will help you "find the love," and keep you from feeling overwhelmed, tired, and resentful while cooking. You will start to notice, as I did, that a meal cooked with love and calm will impact how you metabolize that meal in a more positive manner. You will become more motivated to continue cooking simple meals at home because you will see that this investment will pay you back in energy and contentment.

Harmonious Tip:

Remember that eating food provides nourishment to the body, but preparing it is nourishment for the soul. I love this quote by Elsa Schiaparelli: "A good cook is like a sorcerer who dispenses happiness." Relax, breathe, and plan in advance when you can so that you can more thoroughly enjoy the cooking process and add prana to your food. Don't forget my final tip—the person who does the cooking should not be the one who does the clean up!!

EXPERIMENT WITH NEW TASTES

One of the primary concepts taught by the Institute for Integrative Nutrition is bio-individuality which recognizes that there is no perfect way of eating that works for everyone. One man's food is another man's poison. That is why I can never understand diet programs that preach a defined program that will work for anyone who tries it. We all have different lifestyles, metabolisms, ancestry, blood types, and stress levels, all of which affect what type of foods we should and should not eat. My favorite stage in the coaching process is when my clients finally start to get in tune with their bodies and begin to recognize how the foods they are consuming are affecting all aspects of their life including their energy, mood, and digestion.

Ayurveda is a Sanskrit word derived from spiritual texts from ancient India which means the "knowledge or science of life." I became very interested in learning about Ayurveda while in nutrition school because I found that many Ayurvedic concepts reinforce bio-individuality. I found this fascinating. A book I love about Ayurveda cooking is titled *Eat, Taste, Heal,* which is both a guidebook about Ayurveda wisdom and a cookbook with fabulous recipes. The book discusses the concepts of Ayurveda and explains, "Health is a continuous and participatory process that embraces all aspects of life: physical, mental, emotional behavioral, spiritual, familial, social and universal. Achieving balance on all levels of being is the true measure of vibrant health. Every individual is one-of-a-kind with a unique blueprint for health." When you begin to invest and participate in the process of regaining your health, you stop listening to messages coming from outside and you start to hear your own voice directing you about what your body needs to feel good. You develop a sense of trust in yourself that leads to a certain confidence because you start making decisions that lead you to feel better, and the better you feel, the more you want to continue along this new healthy path.

Learning to understand your own bio-individual way of eating is a very important first step toward a healthy lifestyle and gives you the confidence to be the "expert" about your body. You will stop relying on the media or fad diet books, and trust your own instincts with regard to what you should and should not eat. What I love about this concept is that it allows people to be their own detective about their body and mind in order to make positive food and lifestyle choices. Learning to eat more or less of certain types of foods depending on how you feel is the true definition of taking charge of your health.

To help you become more aware of how certain foods affect you, a great place to begin is by trying new foods and eating a varied diet. In general, Ayurveda recommends eating a balance of all of the six tastes—sweet, sour, salty, bitter, pungent, and astringent.

Sweet foods include grains, pasta, dairy, bread, ripe fruit, and root vegetables which become sweet when cooked. Sweet foods can help calm us when not eaten in excess. Sour foods include citrus fruits such as lemons, oranges, berries, and fermented foods such as vinegar and wine. Sour foods help us to absorb the minerals in our food and can help us to better digest our foods. Salty foods, in addition to any type of salt, include sea vegetables, fish, and meats. Salty foods can stimulate our appetite. Bitter foods include leafy green vegetables like kale and spinach, and vegetables like bell peppers, broccoli, and celery. Some bitter herbs include cilantro, cumin, dill, and turmeric. Bitter foods are wonderful for detoxifying the body. Pungent foods include onions, garlic, and ginger. Pungent spices include basil and thyme. Pungent foods can help clear our nasal passages and help us perspire, reduce inflammation, and aid in digestion. Astringent foods include beans, mushrooms, coffee, and tea. The best way to describe the astringent taste is one that makes your mouth pucker and creates dryness in your mouth. Astringent foods are dehydrating and drying and can be somewhat cooling. These foods can aid in healing.

As I learned more about the different tastes and the effects they have on my body and mind, I began to truly understand how to use food as medicine to heal my body and mind. Learning more about Ayurveda also helped me to better understand how my body's needs vary with the seasons, my stress levels, and my energy expenditure.

The typical American palate has become used to three basic tastes—sweet, sour, and salty. These have become the tastes we crave. Try to begin to incorporate the other three tastes into your cooking and notice the effect they have on you. If you eat out on occasion, experiment with going to an Indian restaurant as their cooking often incorporates all six tastes into each meal. You may feel more satisfied after meals and experience less cravings by adding in some of these unique tastes. See which ones you like, how they make your body feel, and if you enjoy them, increase them in your diet over time.

Harmonious Tip:

You do not need to invest a lot of money to try to incorporate new tastes into your cooking. You can purchase a tiny quantity of a spice before investing in a large bottle in case you find that spice does not work for you. Try adding a few tablespoons of turmeric, cumin, or ginger to your grains and begin experimenting with these new flavors.

SIMPLE MEALS IN NEXT TO NO TIME

I spoke to many people while doing research as I developed my health coaching program and a topic that constantly came up was the challenge of cooking at home. Can you relate to any of these responses?

"I have no free time, no time to cook, and no time to exercise. I want to eat better and cook. I feel fat and uncomfortable."

"I buy ingredients at the store but they often go to waste and I get discouraged. By the time I get home from work or picking up the kids, I am so tired and don't feel like cooking, so I order in food or just eat cereal for dinner. "

"I have trouble cooking at home. It takes too much time. The last thing I want to do after work is come home and cook. I am so hungry when I get home I usually just bring in takeout, but it gets expensive."

We often feel too busy to cook so we rely on takeout food or dine-in restaurants. Sometimes, we even carefully choose the restaurant so that we make "healthy" choices. We justify the expense of takeout food because our time is valuable and we need to eat. I have been there and I know all the justifications. When I lived in New York, the hubby and I would order takeout Chinese food on our commute home from work a couple of times a week. It was a skill we developed—to know exactly when during our commute home we should make the call to our friendly neighborhood Chinese restaurant for delivery so the food would arrive just as we were taking our coats off. We'd think, "Well, it has vegetables in it so it is pretty healthy."

When I began to have health issues, most notably fatigue, brain fog, anxiety and terrible aches and pains in my legs and shoulders, I never suspected that the problem lay in my "healthy" takeout food. I always just assumed the problem was with me. I felt like I needed to calm down, I needed to get it together, think clearer, get organized, and plan my meals. I needed to work out more so I wouldn't be so sore and achy and have headaches. It was during my time studying in nutrition school that I finally made the connection. I looked back at that time in my life and realized the problem did not lay in me, but in the food I was eating. The problem was at the end of my chopsticks!

When we prepare our food at home, we can control the ingredients that go into our meals and we know what we are eating. When we are too busy to cook and we rely on takeout food or restaurant dining, we are at the mercy of the chefs in the kitchen and the large corporations that choose the quality of our ingredients. Looking back, I am sure the Chinese takeout food we were bringing in was loaded with added sugars and salt in quantities I would never use if I were cooking at home. As I learned more about the connection between gluten and the digestive process, I began to understand how all of that soy sauce loaded with MSG and gluten was negatively affecting me. Additionally, restaurants are in business to make a profit so they are buying ingredients with cost in mind. What type of cooking oils are they using? When we cook at home we can choose a good quality cooking oil that fits our budget, but when we eat out, we are subject to whatever oil is least expensive and easiest to cook with but not often the healthiest choice.

Where is your prepared food coming from? Do the sauces and breads have added sugars in them? Are the vegetables organic? Are the meats grass-fed? When we are too busy to cook at home, we have to be very careful where we are getting our meals from. When we are too busy to cook at home, we run the risk of developing health conditions because we can't control everything that is going into our meal. I encourage my clients to speak up and request sauces on the side when they eat out or bring prepared food into their homes. Do not be afraid to tell the restaurant any special dietary needs you have so that if you must eat out you are getting it prepared exactly how you want it.

When I work with clients in my health coaching program, I encourage and support them to get back into the kitchen and try to cook a few simple meals a week at home. I encourage them to find recipes with five ingredients or less. The idea is that the recipes should be high in nutritional value, but not be difficult, complicated, or involve numerous steps and ingredients. I often post simple, delicious recipes on my website like salmon sprinkled with lemon juice, salt, pepper, and dill. I know you are busy, but just getting to the grocery store, prepping, and preparing the meal is the goal. There is no need to be fancy or complex. When you attempt complex recipes on a busy schedule, that is when you get discouraged and decide it is easier to go out to eat. A simple meal with fresh ingredients prepared at home is always better than a fast meal out that is made with poor quality ingredients, oils, and loaded with salt and sugar.

Harmonious Tip:

This week, make a plan to cook a meal once, but eat it several times. That way, you will ensure a healthy meal for your family for at least two nights without expending extra energy on the second night. It seems just as easy to prepare a double or triple batch of something as it is to prepare a single batch, and this will save you time in the long run on the second day or even the third.

FAIL TO PLAN OR PLAN TO FAIL

Oh, that disappointment at the end of a week when you go through the refrigerator and discard any unused produce that has gone bad. The rubbery, flimsy celery, the black bananas, the wilted greens! We hate it because we know it was a waste of money spent on groceries and energy spent shopping.

While an organized, clutter-free kitchen will help with this situation because you will be able to easily spot what you have in your fridge or pantry, the real key is to prep your produce in advance. I always tell my clients, "Fail to plan and plan to fail." I find the best time for me to prep my fruits and veggies is on the weekend when I get home from the grocery store and unpack prior to putting everything in the refrigerator. Others like to prep during the week when they are already cooking in the kitchen, waiting for something to heat up in the oven.

Wash your fruits, cut up your melons, chop your celery, tear and wash your leafy greens, and dice your onions. Doing this in advance will pay you back many times over during the week. First of all, when you get home at the end of the day and need to munch on something immediately, you will have healthy veggies ready to grab and dip into some hummus while you prepare dinner. Second, in the rush of the morning frenzy, you can grab some of these items and quickly pack them up to take for lunch or a snack. Last, when you are tired and have to pull dinner together quickly, just knowing that the onions are diced and the veggies are already washed and prepped will save you loads of time and energy, and motivate you to get dinner on the table.

I also like to prepare my grains on the weekends. I will cook a few cups of brown rice and quinoa, which saves me loads of time during the week. All I have to do is sauté my already chopped onions, add some spices or broth to my grains, and they are ready to eat in no time. I often roast a large chicken on Sunday so I have my protein ready to go during the week. Sometimes I will even roast a tray of vegetables to toss into dinner or bring as a weekday snack in place of raw vegetables.

Sometimes, when I am preparing dinner, I use the time while the water is boiling to pack up my snacks for the next day. The key is to pack your snacks while you are already preparing and cooking other food so that you have everything out on the counter to use, such as your knives and your cutting boards. I also fill up my water bottles for the next day while I am making dinner and pack other snacks such as dried fruit, nuts, and seeds. Avoid the late afternoon problem of grabbing junk food from a vending machine. When you are hungry, your blood sugar will drop, and your brain will start screaming, I NEED FOOD NOW. Be prepared with healthy snacks from home right at your desk or in your car.

Harmonious Tip:

Get some small to medium-sized glass containers with covers that you can fill up with fresh chopped veggies and fruits. Take these with you to work or when you run errands and need a quick, healthy snack. I like to keep a small cooler bag and ice pack that these containers will easily fit into for transporting during warmer weather. You will save time, save money, and save yourself from eating crappy snacks that make you feel like crap. Be prepared so you won't be tempted by the doughnuts in the breakroom at work or the unhealthy snacks at your next meeting!

INVEST IN SOME KITCHEN GADGETS AND USE THEM

I caution you to stay very focused on your kitchen environment when I say this because, as discussed in the Home Environment section, you DO NOT want to clutter up your kitchen. The following are some kitchen tools that have completely changed what and how I cook. They have helped me to enjoy the cooking process more and they save me time.

A CROCKPOT

If you do nothing else that my book suggests, please go out and buy yourself the best crockpot your budget can afford. This is the most wonderful item for the busy, time starved person looking to improve their health. Fill the crockpot the night before with your prepped raw veggies, some spices, a can of broth or salsa, some protein, and a grain. In the morning, plug it in. I always joke that when I arrive home and smell food cooking in the crockpot I feel as though someone else prepared dinner for me. There are tons of simple recipes you can find with a short list of ingredients that will make healthy and delicious meals in the crockpot and I also share some on my website.

SHARP KNIVES

I recently had my entire knife set sharpened, and I was amazed at how much faster my meal preparation went. DO NOT underestimate the value of a sharp knife. It can be one of your greatest time savers, and it will make chopping your fruits and vegetables so much better and simpler and will add to your enjoyment. Keeping your knives sharp will also make for much safer food preparation because a dull knife can slip off the food and hit your fingers. You can learn to sharpen your own knives, or you can have a sharpening service do it for you for a few dollars per knife.

A simple way to check if your knife is sharp is to take a sheet of paper and see if the knife can cleanly cut through the paper as you hold it perpendicular to the papers edge. If you need to use a sawing motion, that means your knife is not sharp enough. You can prolong the sharpness of your knives so you do not have to spend as much time sharpening them if you store them carefully in a block, on a magnetic strip, or in a knife bag and hand wash them instead of putting them in the dishwasher.

A BLENDER

There is a tremendous range of blenders available to fit various budgets and space requirements. My favorite thing to make in the blender is a smoothie for breakfast in the morning. Try to find one that has a single serve attachment so you can throw all your ingredients in, blend them up, and take it on the go. Having a smoothie in the morning is a great way to add greens to your diet. A great time saving tip is to prepare small individual smoothie bags on the weekend to make the morning process simpler. I fill individual Ziploc bags with some berries, a banana, a tablespoon of nut butter and chia seeds, and a couple of handfuls of spinach and store them in the freezer. In the morning, I just empty the Ziploc bag into my blender and add my liquid, usually some almond or coconut milk, and blend. This is a great way to get your kids to eat breakfast as well.

AN IMMERSION BLENDER

My immersion blender has elevated my soups to a whole new level that I did not expect. The simple act of partially blending a portion of your pot of soup gives the soup a whole different taste and texture that is wonderful. An immersion blender is a handheld blender that you immerse into a large pot which can puree and liquefy whatever you are blending.

My lentil soups are much more savory since blending them. I have prepared corn soup that becomes creamy and full of flavor. I have even prepared squash soup with the immersion blender. You can find these blenders in stores at varying price points, but you can spend under $50 like I did and have great results. I find that soup is a great timesaver because you can prepare a large pot on the weekend and package it up in individual containers for the week. Because soup freezes very well, it is great to keep some containers in your freezer for busy evenings where only one person in the family will be eating at home.

If you are not ready to invest in a blender, your immersion blender can also serve to prepare individual smoothies, and it is very quick and easy to clean.

PREP AND WASTE BOWLS

I used to watch the cooking shows on TV where they used these tiny bowls to measure out the herbs and spices in advance but never thought to try it at home. When I invested in some very small prep bowls, I noticed how much simpler meal preparation became. When you begin to plan in advance, another big time saver is to premeasure your spices. I found some small prep bowls with covers that I now use to measure the spices and herbs out in advance. This saves so much time when you are cooking, and lets you enjoy the process so much more because you don't have to worry that something will burn while you are digging around in the pantry for the turmeric or the cinnamon and trying to find your measuring spoons.

Cooking with a waste bowl will save you tons of time during clean up. A waste bowl is just any medium to large sized bowl placed on the counter next to you in which you put onion skins, melon rinds, egg shells, chicken fat, or even to use as a place to rest a dirty spoon. Your counter will require less cleanup and you won't have to make several trips to the trash can—just one at the end to discard the contents of the bowl.

Harmonious Tip:

Do not clutter up your kitchen with gadgets you likely will use once and never use again. Invest some time walking through a kitchen store or shopping online and see if there are any tools or gadgets that might inspire you to start cooking more or that save you some time. But please, whatever you do, go buy a crockpot. If you have one at home that you have forgotten about, pull it out of the closet and start using it again!

5

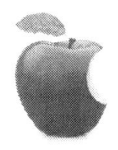

Healthy Mind

"Whether you think you can or think you can't, you're right."

- Henry Ford

Prior to adopting Harmonious Health habits, my evenings were often wrecked by my conditioned response to react to the normal "chaos" that ensued when I got home and the kids were done with school. Last minute realizations that the science assignment was due tomorrow and poster board was needed ASAP would put me in a tizzy. The barking dog, the phone ringing, the spilled juice all over the floor, and the stack of mail with the bills glaring at me right on top started to make me want to forget about my all-day efforts to be healthy and grab a bag of potato chips and go hide under the covers.

As I began to practice what I was learning, incorporated journaling into my routine, and truly internalized and valued the importance of being in nature and scheduling time for that in my daily routine, I noticed that my poor conditioned responses to the chaos and stress going on in my home in the evenings went away. Yes, I was still busy, and yes, I still knew someone needed to go to Target and buy the poster board, even though it was late and I was tired, but knowing I had an appointment that night with myself and my bubble bath helped me to remain composed, and not let my stress response get the best of me. Practicing deep breathing exercises for just five minutes kept me grounded and helped me to gain a more realistic perspective on situations, which ultimately saved me time and wasted energy. The result was a happier, calmer me, and happier, less guilt-ridden kids, a better relationship with the hubby, and to my surprise, more productivity for me. Focusing on the primary foods in my life (my relationships, my happiness, my spirituality) helped me live a calmer, more productive life with more grace and ease.

Taking better control over my thoughts even helped me to better manage my cravings. When I went out to Target to buy the poster board, instead of grabbing a candy bar at the checkout, my calmer, clearer thinking reminded me that I was out of organic spinach which I needed for my morning smoothie the next day. My calmer demeanor helped me think better, and I stopped wasting time complaining about petty things during the day because this new attitude was helping me to improve my relationships and to become a more forgiving and understanding person. I came to realize it was not TIME that was challenging me, it was my response to my perceived limited free time that was the challenge. Once I changed my response, I seemed to find more hours of productivity in my day, and less time for stress and worry.

As I spent more time in nature, I was more interested in meal planning and had a better appreciation for my food. I was finding inspiration for cooking during my quiet moments outdoors, and making a connection between nature and my food. Subsequently, when I would cook, I felt calmer and happier because somehow the cooking process, chopping fresh herbs or massaging my kale, reconnected me with the happiness I felt when I was spending time outdoors.

NO TIME TO THINK? USE A JOURNAL

When I work with new clients, I always give them a journal at our first session and ask them to keep track of what they are eating and how they are feeling. In the beginning, people are very excited to write down everything they eat and stay very on top of this exercise. It helps them connect the food they are eating to how they are feeling and the effect it is having on their moods. This is a great tool to identify a bio-individual nutrition plan that is right for them.

As time goes by and they make progress in this area, I then ask them to use the journal in whatever way works for them, but to try to keep track of any changes or small steps they are taking to improve their health each day. I have them jot down things like, "Drank an extra cup of water before lunch," or, "Added extra veggies to my dinner last night," or, "Did a few stretches this morning before my shower." Keeping track of the small steps helps them to focus on the changes they are making rather than the results. When people focus on results only, they can get very discouraged, but focusing on the changes they are making helps keep them stay motivated and productive. I love this quote by Jack Dixon: "If you focus on results, you will never change. If you focus on change, you will get results."

Julia Cameron, author of *The Writer's Way*, talks about an exercise called "morning pages" in which you write about everything on your mind when you first wake up in the morning. Her idea is that by emptying your head of all your fears, worries, and thoughts first thing in the morning, you then free your mind to focus on the tasks that lay ahead of you and can more easily flow through your day. There is no outline or format for how to do this, just free flowing thoughts written on the page. For some people, morning pages works, while for others, getting into bed at the end of the evening and emptying all of their thoughts onto paper then helps them to unwind and clear their head. Whatever time of day works for you, give journaling a try.

I was a bit skeptical when I first started journaling, but the more I practiced, the more I enjoyed it, and here I am now, writing my very first book. Journaling can help the everyday busy person to organize their thoughts, which over time, can save hours of confusion and discomfort. There is no way to tell how journaling will affect you personally, but I guarantee if you give it a try, at the very least, it can help slow your mind down, help you unwind from being on the go, and identify what thoughts are on your mind which can help stifle any anxiety you may be experiencing. Allow yourself an opportunity to relax and unwind. Try not to view this exercise as another "to do" on your list that eats up your time. Through journaling, I have resolved issues, noticed trends about foods that were making me feel poorly, and found it to be an unexpected form of relaxation.

Harmonious Tip:

Treat yourself to a unique notebook or a bound journal with an inspirational cover. Grab a special pen and start experimenting with getting your thoughts on paper. Express gratitude for someone special in your life. Make a list of five wonderful things that make you happy, or jot down one or two goals. Give it a try and you just might discover a newfound, unexpected pleasure.

REMEMBER TO BREATHE

Years ago, I had an awesome Pilates instructor who pointed out to me that during the difficult parts of the class, I would hold my breath. I mistakenly believed that holding my breath would somehow help me fight through the tough parts of the class. When I started to take deep breaths and exhale loudly, I was amazed at how much more effective I was at completing the exercises and how much easier it was to hold a pose. I noticed how breathing into the pain helped to ease it.

While deep breathing, of course, has profound, positive effects on your body, I include it here, in mind habits, because during tense and stressful moments of your day, deep breathing can help you relax your mind and help you regain composure and perspective. Your mind cannot be troubled when your breathing is regular and calm. You can immediately influence your emotional state by consciously breathing in a controlled way.

In nutrition school, Dr. Andrew Weil taught us a deep belly breathing technique known as "4-7-8 breathing" that has helped me and many of my clients to slow down during the day and regroup. The wonderful thing about this exercise is you can do it anywhere and anytime you need it. The technique is based on Pranayama, which is an ancient Indian practice. To practice the "4-7-8 breathing" technique, first exhale completely through your mouth. Then, close your mouth and inhale quietly through your nose to a count of four. Now, hold your breath for a count of seven. Next, exhale completely through your mouth for eight seconds in one large breath. Now, inhale again through your nose, and repeat the cycle three times for a total of four breaths. Keep the tip of your tongue where your two front teeth meet your gums during the exercise.

Whenever you feel tense during the day, rather than reaching for a sugary or salty treat or a caffeinated beverage, try this natural breathing technique instead to allow your mind to relax and to reduce the tension in your body.

Harmonious Tip:

Try to practice the "4-7-8 deep belly breathing" exercise twice a day, and over time, you will begin to establish a wonderful habit. Shallow breathing does not allow your body to get the amount of oxygen it needs. By practicing deep belly breathing, you improve your digestion and circulation, you can slow down a rapid heart rate, slow the release of toxins, and calm your mind. Breathing will help you relax during the day or before bed, release tension, and can bring new clarity and insight to your thoughts.

FOCUS ON YOUR PRIMARY FOOD

One of the concepts that distinguishes my health coaching program from other programs is the idea of primary food. You will not see primary food on the USDA MyPlate. You will not hear diet centers or other programs that sell pills and powders for weight loss talk about primary food, which is one of the reasons these weight loss programs do not really help people in the long term. In order to make permanent changes to your secondary food (the food you eat), you must address your primary food. Primary foods include your relationships, career satisfaction, spirituality, and exercise.

When I first began health coaching, I did not expect to be discussing these areas of my client's lives with them, but it is during these conversations that I see some of the biggest breakthroughs. I encourage my clients to look at these four aspects of their lives as a form of nutrition because these aspects of life "feed" them on a much deeper level than food does. The food we eat plays a central role in creating our health and wellness, and it is extremely important for us to discover the right foods for our unique bodies. However, the four forms of primary food nourish us by making our lives complete and wonderful when combined with a healthy food plan.

When our primary foods are balanced and satisfying, our life fills us up with joy, it "feeds" us. Our hunger for the food we eat diminishes as we feel "full" in our soul, and the physical food we eat becomes "secondary food." How does a busy person lose balance in their primary foods? In an article in The Economist, *In Search of Lost Time; Why Is Everyone so Busy?:*

> "When people are paid more to work, they tend to work longer hours because working becomes a more profitable use of time. So the rising value of work time puts pressure on all time. Leisure time starts to seem more stressful as people feel compelled to use it wisely or not at all."
>
> (The Economist. In Search of Lost Time; Why Is Everyone so Busy? The Economist. Print Edition. The Economist Newspaper Limited, 20 Dec. 2014)

It is interesting to me that analysis of time stress data found that those with bigger paychecks felt more anxiety about their time.

It often seems that time is most valued once it is gone. Yet we continue to hurry, to rush, to not be present. Why are people doing this? Maybe we are trying to avoid certain feelings, and if we constantly stay busy, we distract ourselves from deep feelings that cause us disease and make us feel bad. Focusing on your primary foods takes effort because you have to be mindful and that requires a certain degree of energy and awareness.

Just like our eating habits, rushing around and constantly feeling like you don't have enough time is a habit, and just like a sugar habit, it becomes addicting.

Ask yourself the following questions to see if your primary foods are in balance:

1. Are my relationships with my spouse, children, other family members, friends, and coworkers healthy and do they support my individual wants and needs?

2. Is physical activity a habit that I fit into my weekly schedule?

Different types of movement nourish our bodies in various ways. I work with my clients to help them identify what form will keep them feeling balanced, nourish them, and fit into their schedule. Some of my clients who have been rigorously doing intense aerobic exercise several days a week begin to substitute one day a week with light stretching or yoga. This change helps them in unexpected ways because the intensity of too much aerobic activity was making them very stressed by increasing their cortisol levels. When they substitute a softer exercise one day a week, they notice they have less food cravings because they feel less tight and tense, and are more easily able to lose weight. Ask yourself if your current exercise routine fits your current condition based on your schedule, state of mind, and the time and energy demands being put on you. Adjust as needed.

3. I spend eight to ten hours a day at work—am I doing work that I love?

Maybe you need a new career if the answer is, "No." Maybe you just need a change in your workspace environment, a raise, a more flexible work schedule, or just a conversation with your supervisor. Go after whatever you need to make your job a more positive experience. I do not think it is a coincidence that two of my recent clients in my six-month coaching program switched jobs while we worked together as they began to focus on their primary foods. As a result, they felt happier and had more energy to devote to other aspects of their lives, which positively impacted their health.

4. Do you have a spiritual practice that adds meaning to your life? Does it help take you away from focusing on material things and your physical self by connecting you on a deeper level to your human soul or spirit?

For some people, this is practicing their religion. For others, it is a hobby or other form or meditation. Having a spiritual practice that is part of your life on a regular basis will help you cope with the normal ups and downs that we all experience and will bring you more happiness.

Harmonious Tip:

It is helpful to sit down once in a while and reflect on the various parts of your life, your career, exercise routines, relationships, spirituality, and examine how satisfied you are in each of these areas. This will help you to understand where you should focus your time to improve your happiness, which will ultimately bring more joy and better health to your overall life. People often spend a lot of time exerting energy on something they think will bring them joy, but when they sit down and reevaluate the various areas of their life, they realize that this is not an area they should be investing so much energy and time in.

TAKE TIME FOR NATURE

I can remember spending several weeks in the summer at a sleep away camp as a child. I spent most of my time outdoors, woke up to crisp east coast mornings, spent warm days in the lake, and breathed in cool evening air. When I sent my own kids off to summer camp, I noticed them returning with that same carefree, calm happiness that I'd felt each summer. While I understood that a large part of this attitude had to do with the fact that there was no schoolwork, homework, or pressure, as I began to learn more about the health benefits of spending time in nature, I realized that this is also what contributed to that lighthearted, carefree mood.

I love this quote from Samuel Johnson: "Deviation from nature is deviation from happiness." In our hi-tech society, many people are suffering from what is being called "Nature Deficit Disorder," which is spending way too much time indoors, away from fresh air and natural beauty. While it is always great to bring plants and other elements of nature into our homes, nothing feels quite the same as spending good quality time outdoors.

Researchers in the field of ecotherapy, also known as green therapy, which means improving your mental and physical wellbeing through outdoor activities in nature, are finding that spending time in nature can help alleviate symptoms of depression. In addition to helping lift depression, being in nature, even for as little as twenty minutes, can improve your energy. Like Johnson's quote says, being in nature is linked to happiness. I bet you are thinking, "Great, but I am busy, Suzy, and I don't have time to just sit around and hang out in nature. I don't have time to go for a long hike in the woods." Okay, I get it. The weekdays are rough, but do you have some phone calls you have to return? Consider making them on your cell phone while you take the dog for a walk. Have some unanswered work emails you didn't get to? Can you bring your laptop outside and sit in your backyard or terrace or on a folding chair and answer them? Do you have kids you need to pick up at an activity? Can you arrive a few minutes in advance, and instead of sitting in your car mindlessly wasting time on Facebook, can you park the car and walk around the soccer field or outside the gym while you wait for them?

The Jewish holiday of Sukkot usually falls around late September, early October. During this holiday, we eat outdoors in nature in a walled structure called a sukkah covered with plant materials such as palm leaves. It marks the end of harvest time in Israel and the sukkah serves as a reminder of the fragile structures the Israelites lived in during the forty years they wandered and survived after the exodus from Egypt. I always feel so happy during this week, being outside, eating my meals in nature. The summer has been over for several weeks, school is back in session, and it is a great reminder to get back outside and notice the changing of the season. Why not bring your meals outside throughout the year, weather permitting? Just grab your dinner plate and enjoy the beauty of the evening and the twinkling stars. You are busy, but you still have to eat, so move that meal outside and get the double benefit of the nutrition on your plate while being nurtured by nature at the same time.

Harmonious Tip:

Choose an outdoor environment this week by your office or your home and take a slow walk around it, noticing what you see, smell, hear, and can touch. Doing this will put you more in touch with the seasons, give you a greater appreciation for the seasonal food you eat, and make you feel more connected to the earth. The more time you spend in nature, the more you will notice yourself making choices about sustainable living and supporting environmental causes. As you begin to appreciate the benefits you feel from our planet, you will be inspired to take better care of it. I have even noticed myself feeling better when I am wearing clothing made of 100% natural fabrics, which gives me a greater feeling of connectedness to the earth. Schedule time right now into your week where you can devote even just ten minutes to being in nature. As you notice its positive affect on you, you will be motivated to schedule more and more time for nature.

GIVE YOUR CRAVINGS THE TIME OF DAY

I considered including this section of the book in the eating section. After all, our cravings obviously affect what we decide to eat. After careful consideration of the numerous conversations I have had with clients and friends, I realized that it really belongs here. Cravings take a toll on our emotional state of mind, and what I recently noticed is it takes a toll on a woman's self-esteem. Over and over again I hear women tell me, "I was bad this week," or, "I had no self-control," or, "I f***ed up," or, "I suck, I can't stick with anything."

A great tool I share with my clients is teaching them how to deconstruct their cravings, meaning getting to the root of what is causing them. Over the period of time I work with my clients, we discuss triggers to cravings and set up systems to help them avoid these triggers. We also look at deficiencies that may be causing these triggers, both in their primary and secondary foods.

Here are just a few tips on how to do this:

Drink Water - One of the best things to do when you get a craving is to first drink a full glass of water. Sometimes we are just thirsty and this will satisfy us. Eating when we are not truly hungry compromises and overloads our digestive system. So grab a glass of water to start.

Understand What Your Body Needs - After drinking the water, if you still have an overwhelming desire to raid the pantry for something you know you should not eat, take a moment to think about what it is that your body needs. We can't ignore cravings, they won't go away, and they will always win. Cravings are controlled in your brain and they signal to the body what you might be deficient in. Cravings are your body's natural way of surviving by telling you what nutrients and minerals you might need.

For Sweet Cravings - If you are craving sweets, try to first satisfy this with a food that does not contain refined white sugar. Try eating a date, a piece of an apple, or a banana first. Food prepared or topped with natural sweeteners like raw wild honey, coconut nectar, or pure maple syrup are other good alternatives. Eating lots of whole foods, especially cooked sweet vegetables like corn, carrots, onions, beets, squash, and sweet potatoes can help reduce sweet cravings. When these veggies are cooked, they develop a sweet flavor that satisfies you the more you eat them. If you must satisfy your sweet craving with chocolate, choose the best quality you can find for the money and eat it and enjoy it slowly. You will find this much more satisfying than inhaling a bag of M&M's, especially because you will not be filled with guilt afterward.

For Salt Cravings - Frequently craving salt? You might be deficient in minerals so eating leafy green veggies high in minerals can help. I also suggest replacing your white table sale with a high quality sea salt, rich in minerals (my favorite is pink Himalayan sea salt). Also try adding sea vegetables to your meals. To satisfy a salt craving quickly, pop your own organic popcorn kernels, season with some lovely pink Himalayan salt, and add in some hot sauce.

Craving Something Crispy - Try to avoid processed chips and crackers loaded with artificial ingredients, and instead, choose healthier versions with high quality ingredients you can pronounce like rice cakes, five ingredients or less crackers, or sugar-free sesame sticks. Sometimes munching on celery or a handful of nuts can settle a craving for crispy. If you are feeling adventurous, thinly slice a potato, spray with olive oil, sprinkle with salt, and bake in the oven until crispy.

Harmonious Tip:

The main thing is to not ignore your cravings or to be frustrated with yourself for having them, but to learn what it is your body is trying to tell you. Often times, what you need is not food, but rest, fresh air, movement, or stress relief. In my six-month program, I teach clients how to distinguish what it is their body needs, which leads to less guilt, less stress, better energy and focus throughout the day, and less bloating and other discomforts caused by giving in to cravings in the wrong way. Spending a few minutes trying to understand your cravings before you give in to them will help you to feel better later on.

MEAL PLANNING

I believe in positive thinking, goal setting, visualizing your success, and having an attitude of gratitude. I love coaching clients to use these techniques in their daily lives.

I believe all of these techniques will lead to greater satisfaction, contentment, confidence, and happiness in our lives, and I practice all of these techniques in my daily life. I read about them, I listen to audios, and watch videos on all of these topics so that I can further develop and strengthen all these skills and coach my clients on them.

However, after working with many women who were looking to improve their health and wellness, I have found that if peace does not exist in their minds around meal planning, no amount of positive thinking, goal setting, or any other self-help technique will bring them happiness and contentment.

So what is it about meal planning that makes some people cringe with pain, while others would not dare end their Sunday without a full week of meals planned out?
Just merely asking several women and getting the initial response was informative.

"What is your process around meal planning?" I asked. I got a lot of sighs, laughs, moans, and some excitement. The one thing in common, however, was the sentiment that if I plan my meals ahead of time, my entire week goes so much smoother.

People are searching for the perfect meal planning system and constantly criticizing themselves for not having one. They're frustrated by their attempts to try, so they give up. Human nature also causes many to use the little free time they do have in ways that seem more thrilling than planning meals and grocery shopping. But truth be told, as I mentioned earlier, fail to plan and you will plan to fail.

I wish I could tell you I have a solid strategy in place around my meal planning, but I do not. It varies from week to week. I read blogs, I follow some Instagram and Facebook accounts for recipe and meal plan ideas, I read cookbooks constantly, and I use some meal planning apps. The one constant I do have each week is that I make sure that before I go to bed on Sunday night, I have a plan for at least three weekday meals that I will cook, and that I have the necessary grocery items in the house needed to prepare them. In addition, I always make sure I have emergency staple items on hand.

Some staples you will always find in my kitchen include bags of frozen organic vegetables and berries, onions, garlic, cans of beans, dried rice, quinoa, oats, frozen meats, cooking oils, spices, vinegar, diced tomatoes, nuts and seeds, lemon or lime juice, honey, vanilla, eggs, nut butters, almond milk, cacao powder, and dark chocolate. As long as I have these items on hand, it seems I can always find a way to come up with a breakfast, lunch, or dinner and some satisfying snacks.

I find that it is very tempting to prepare meals that I am familiar with and do not require a recipe for because it makes life much easier. The problem with this strategy is that I noticed I would continually cook the same meals over and over again, which creates boredom, and less mealtime satisfaction. In addition, I learned that sometimes we develop food sensitivities if we eat the same food over and over again. Eating a varied diet is best so that you cover all different nutritional bases and you're not getting too much of one thing. For weekday recipes, I try to use recipes with no more than five ingredients to keep it simple

Here is some advice to help the busy person plan their meals. Each week, decide on one main meal you would enjoy for the upcoming week and think about how that meal's protein is prepared. Is it cooked in a crockpot, cooked on the stovetop in a frying pan, baked in the oven, or boiled in a pot on the stove? I have found that just considering how the food will be cooked and alternating it weekly helps me think quickly about what I will be preparing. If I have not baked in the oven much the prior week, I will think trays or roasted vegetables or pieces of chicken or fish baked with a nice sauce. If I have not used my big soup pot in a while, I will think veggie chili, meatballs in a sauce, or a nice and tasty lentil soup. If the crockpot needs to come out, I think delicious stew, chicken on the bone cooked in tomato sauce, or a whole chicken with veggies cooked for hours into a gut healthy bone broth. For my big wok style frying pan, I think veggie stir fry, black bean burgers, sautéed spiralized vegetables. For my long rectangular Pyrex dish, I think veggie lasagna. For my small frying pan, I think veggie egg frittata. While your own personal meal preferences will vary, I have found this to be a quick and easy way to think about meal planning. Then, on the weekend, take that big pot, pan, or crockpot out and set it on the kitchen stovetop.

Now that you have a plan, on the weekend or one evening, go in your pantry for the non-perishables. What will you need for that meal that would be in the pantry? Beans, pasta, rice, quinoa—take it out and place it in that pot, pan, or casserole dish. Next, how will you season it? Take out those spices, take the oil container out of the closet, and put them in that same container. Now take a rest. Just leave that out in the kitchen, let it remind you of what you are planning to cook. Let it motivate you because it is a reminder of the positive steps you have taken toward next week's meal.

Now consider what produce will you need—what meats, fish, eggs, anything that needs refrigeration? Do you have that in the house, in the freezer? If so, take it out of the freezer to thaw. Make a list of what you will need and purchase those items at the store.

Now, here you are, it's Monday night, your meeting ran late, and you are getting home and feeling "hangry." Change into your comfy clothes and grab a glass of water or some herbal tea. The pot is already pulled out, your onions are already chopped, and the oil and the spices are already out of the pantry in the pan. Turn on the cooktop, heat the oil, and sauté the onions with your meat. Play with the spices that you selected. You are actually enjoying this, everything was there waiting for you. You feel like a chef in a fancy cooking school! The sauce is already out so just open it and add it in. You have saved so much time just taking everything out in advance and assembling it in one place that you are actually loving this process. Now you grab those beautiful veggies you cut on the weekend, toss them into the pot, and you feel giddy because this was effortless tonight! You think, "This is fabulous. I can't wait to taste it." You feel energized looking at all of this delicious food cooking in the pot because you barely exerted any energy tonight to pull this masterpiece together. It felt effortless because it was! All of the effort was spread out over the weekend and now you are finally understanding that cooking at home can actually relax you. Congratulations, you are a meal planning master!

Harmonious Tip:

On the weekend, thoroughly read through the recipes you plan to cook during the week to determine what, if any, special tools or cooking equipment you will need in addition to ingredients. Measure out all ingredients before you get started. This one simple step has completely changed how I cook. No more burning onions while fiddling to find other ingredients! You will find that if you get all of your ingredients prepped and measured out before you start, you will also enjoy the cooking process so much more.

CUT TO THE CHASE

Are you racing against time with no time to kill? I know how you feel. I have felt it myself. If only there were more hours in the day. What we really need to do is maximize the productive hours we have in a day by having better energy and focus. By incorporating my Harmonious Habits into your daily routine you will begin to achieve this.

It is time for you to make a change in your attitude about what the real obstacle is, and there is no time like the present. The real obstacle to vibrant health is not a lack of time, but a lack of focused attention on the small changes in habits that you need to make. It is just a matter of time before all of this racing against the clock and ignoring your wellness is going to catch up to you and you will need to carve out large amounts time to address it. Dedicate small amounts of focused attention over the next few weeks to your various habits around eating, cooking, thinking, moving, and your environment so you can avoid the need to lose large amounts of time down the road to potential illness or the side effects that can result from poor nutrition and lifestyle habits.

By following the Harmonious Health tips in my program,

you can simply and easily begin to improve on aspects of your health that will lead to vibrant wellness in next to no time. If you are looking for even more tips and support, contact me to work one-on-one as your health coach in one of my customized programs that is right for you. There is so much information out there regarding diet plans, exercise, and lifestyle habits that it can often be overwhelming. Together, we can create a customized plan that is right for you, for your personal lifestyle, schedule, body, and nutritional needs, one that takes into account your likes and dislikes.

A health coach helps you put the systems in place that will work specifically for your unique self to improve the quality of your life through healthy habits. I will help you to understand why your previous attempts to get healthy may have failed, and I will stick with you to keep you motivated and inspired. The greatest result of working with a health coach is that I will teach you how to rely on yourself. Working together, I will teach you how to trust your body and what it needs so that you can successfully change your habits to achieve your goal of good health. You will no longer feel confused by all of the conflicting nutrition advice you are reading about because you will be the expert, the authority on what your own body needs.

When you choose Harmonious Health as a priority, you will save money on medical bills and you will save time on trips to the doctor. You will have more energy and accomplish more in your day, which will increase your confidence and reduce your stress, allowing you to spend more time with loved ones and pursuing activities you love. This will add to your longevity and deepen your connection to yourself and with others. Rather than addressing your symptoms, we will get to the root cause of what is holding you back from achieving Harmonious Health.

ABOUT THE AUTHOR

Born, raised, and educated in New York, Suzy Harmon toiled in the rat race as a CPA in New York City for many years. She served in a variety of accounting positions including as an auditor at an international public accounting firm, at two major worldwide corporations in the advertising and entertainment industry, and most recently, for small business owners after she and her family moved to Texas.

Family life is something Suzy cherishes, but she also knows what it's like to feel too busy for healthy living. Suzy found herself at a crossroads after seeing people pay extreme prices for professional advancement by letting their health and family lives suffer. Suzy's core insight is that "your greatest wealth is health," and this is what motivated her to change her lifestyle and impart that wisdom to others. Suzy wants her clients to enjoy fabulous health so they can experience the joys of life and the rewards of their hard work for many, many years.

Healthy eating, cooking, exercise, and overall wellbeing have always been Suzy's passion, so she strives to help others who are sacrificing their physical health in search of happiness by arming them with a healthier plan for success.

In January of 2014, Suzy allowed her passion for health to guide her and she became certified as a Health Coach at the Institute for Integrative Nutrition where she was trained in more than one hundred dietary theories and studied a variety of practical lifestyle coaching methods. Drawing on this knowledge, she can now help her clients find the healthy balance they are looking for in all areas of their lives. She helps them create a completely personalized "roadmap to health" that suits their unique body, lifestyle, preferences, and goals.

Empowering others to make healthy food and lifestyle choices that energize their body and enrich their spirit and mind is all part of Suzy's program at Harmonious Health.

To learn more about Suzy and how Harmonious Health can help you take control of a healthy approach to achieving your goals, or to book her for a speaking engagement, visit her website at www.suzyharmonioushealth.com or email Suzy directly at harmonioushealth@sbcglobal.net

Made in the USA
San Bernardino, CA
10 May 2016